FRCR Part 2

MCQs

on

THORACIC RADIOLOGY

AND

CARDIAC RADIOLOGY

DR NAGENDRA KUMAR SINHA

MD (Radio-diagnosis)

Copyright © 2015

Dr. Nagendra Kumar Sinha

All rights reserved.

No part of this publication may be reproduced or transmitted in any form or any means , electronic , mechanical , photocopy , recording, translated ,or any information storage and retrieval system ,without permission in writing from this author.

ISBN-13: **978-1511778121**
ISBN-10: **1511778121**

TO
MY BROTHER
SHYAM KISHOR PRASAD SINHA
AND
SISTER-IN-LAW
MANJULA RANI RENU
FOR THEIR
LOVE AND GUIDANCE

PREFACE

MCQs is a standard format to assess the conceptual and factual knowledge. FRCR has adopted the same approach .This MCQs book on THORACIC AND CARDIAC RADIOLOGY contains 14 TEST PAPERS .Each test paper consists of 50 questions and so this book contains 700 MCQs (14 x50 =700).Each test paper is designed to cover all the different topics of thoracic and cardiac radiolgy.Some of mcqs are deliberately repeated .The each test paper is followed by answer with detailed explanations with reference .Most of MCQs are based on **Adam: Grainger & Allison's Diagnostic Radiology, 5th ed.**

I believe this book will prove to be a perfect revision tool for candidate sitting in the FRCR PART 2A (Thoracic and cardiac radiology).This MCQs book will surely be of great help and guidance for those who aspire to clear the exam of FRCR.
This book will also be useful as a sharpening tool for radiologists and residents and all those doctors who wish to make concept of Thoracic and cardiac radiology more clear.

Wishing you all the best,
Nagendra Kumar Sinha
E-mail:ngdrkus@yahoo.co.in
Blog:nagendra's radiology blog

CONTENTS

Acknowledgments

1.Test paper 1 and answer	7---19
2.Test paper 2 and answer	20---32
3.Test paper 3 and answer	33---44
4.Test paper 4 and answer	45---58
5.Test paper 5 and answer	59---72
6.Test paper 6 and answer	73---86
7.Test paper 7 and answer	87---100
8.Test paper 8 and answer	101--112
9.Test paper 9 and answer	113--124
10.Test paper 10 and answer	125--137
11.Test paper 11 and answer	**138--149**
12.Test paper 12 and answer	**150---161**
13.Test paper 13 and answer	**162---174**
14.Test paper 14 and answer	**175---188**

ACKNOWLEDGEMENTS

I am grateful to ALMIGHTY GOD who inspired and gave me strength to write this book.

I am grateful to my teachers,particularly Dr. N K Gogoi and Dr R K Gogoi, who chided me for my ignorance and prodded me towards excellence,

I am grateful to my father late Dwarika Prasad and mother Smt Kaushalya devi for their constant blessings

I really feel privileged to extend my gratitude to my brother Er S K P Sinha and sister-in law Manjula Rani Renu.

I am grateful to my wife Rina sinha and my son Anmol Kumar Sinha and Rajat Kumar Sinha for sacrifice they made during my engagement . I am highly indebtebted to my father-in-law R A Roy and mother –in law Aruna Roy and sister-in-law Anju Roy and Nina Roy .

I am grateful to my colleagues and seniors for their support ,cooperation and suggestions.

I am grateful to Facebook and Nagendra's radiology blog fraternity who responded and appreciated the questions posted by me during manuscripts preparation.

Special thanks to my friend Sanjay jayaswal and Ashok kumar who is always with me in all time and everytime.

Nagendra Kumar Sinha

TEST PAPER 1

1.All are true regarding diaphragm except
a) the angle of contact with the chest wall is acute and sharp,
b) blunting of CP angle can be normal in athletes
c) the normal right hemidiaphragm is found at about the level of the anterior portion of the sixth rib(+/- approximately one interspace)
d) the right hemidiaphragm is 1.5–2.5 cm higher than the left in most cases
e) the two hemidiaphragms are at the same level in some 19% of the population.

2.Typical X-ray finding of pneumothorax in erect position
a) pleural air in vicinity of the lung apex
b)visceral pleural line
c) a transradiant zone
d)area devoid of vessels
e)the 'pneumothorax' line beyond the margin of the chest cavity

3.Signs of pneumothorax in supine positions are all except
a) ipsilateral transradiancy (generalized or hypochondrial)
b) a deep, finger-like costophrenic sulcus laterally
c) double diaphragm sign and diaphragmatic elevation
d) a transradiant band parallel to the diaphragm and/or mediastinum
e) visualization of the undersurface of the heart, and of the cardiac fat pads

4.All are true regarding mediastinal lymph nodes except
a)Normal sized nodes are not visible on plain chest radiographs
b) Nodes in the right paratracheal group cause uniform or lobular widening of the right paratracheal stripe
c) the lymph nodes in aorto-pulmonary window cause a local bulge in the angle between the aortic arch and the main pulmonary artery.
d) Subcarinal lymph node enlargement cause the subcarinal portion of the azygo-oesophageal line to produce concavity towards the lung,
e) Posterior mediastinal lymph node enlargement causes localized displacement of the paraspinal and para-oesophageal lines

5.All are true regarding sarcoidosis except
a) the most common cause of intrathoracic lymph node enlargement
b)the hilar nodes enlarged in almost all cases in symmetrical way
c) tracheobronchial, aortopulmonary and subcarinal nodes are enlarged in over half the patients
d)Anterior mediastinal nodes occasionally increase in size
e) posterior mediastinal node enlargement is very common

6.All are true regarding post-primary tuberculosis except
a) Most cases are due to reactivation of quiescent lesions
b) arise in the apicoposterior segments of an upper lobe and/or the superior segment of a lower lobe
c) Isolated involvement of the anterior segment of an upper lobe almost diagnostic
d) Cavitation is seen in the region of abnormality in 40–80% of cases
e) A Rasmussen aneurysm complication of cavitary tuberculosis

7.All are true regarding post primary pulmonary tuberculosis after healing except
a. upper lobe nodular and linear opacities
b. obliteration of cavities usual
c. severe volume loss and pleural thickening
d. Bronchiectasis and the formation of cysts and bullae
e. calcification of opacities more common than with primary tuberculosis

8.Emphysema is characterized by all except
a. permanent, abnormal enlargement of airspaces
b. distal to the respiratory bronchioles
c. the destruction of walls of air spaces
d. no obvious fibrosis
e. cigarette smoking most important factor

9.Emphysema is associated with
a. cigarette smoking

b. nitrogen oxides and phosphogenes
c. deficiency of protease
d. cutix laxa
e. Marfan syndrome

10.All are true regading pulmonary neoplasm except
a.most of pulmonary sarcomas are metastatic in natue
b. bronchocentric distribution of the lesions is noted in pulmonary Kaposi Sarcoma
c. The most common malignant tumour of the trachea is invasion from an adjacent neoplasm
d. adenoid cystic carcinomas may calcify
e. Typical carcinoids most commonly arise in central airways

11.All are true regarding bronchial carcinoid except
a. typical carcinoid accounts for 85–90% of bronchial carcinoid
b. Typical carcinoids most commonly arise in central airways.
c.may metastatize
d.iceberg 's lesions noted
e.bronchial carcinoid never calcify

12.All are true regarding interstitial fibrosis except
a. diffuse alveolar damage (DAD) noted in acute interstitial pneumonia
b. acute exudative phase , organizing and fibrotic phase in acute interstitial pneumonia
c. thin-walled cysts (1–30 mm) in LIP
d. Airspace disease, large nodules and pleural effusions common in LIP

e. Intrathoracic Castleman's disease frequently associated with LIP

13.All are true regarding sarcoidosis except

a. Granulomas along the lymphatics in the bronchovascular sheath

b. the most commonly affected organ ---the hilar ,mediastinal nodes and the lungs

c. stage II refers to lymphadenopathy with parenchymal opacity

d. bilateral, symmetrical hilar and paratracheal lymphadenopathy

e. significant compression of adjacent airways, arteries and veins very usual

14.Pneumomediastinum is characterized by all except

a. the visible thymus

b. air posterior to the pericardium

c. air surrounding the pulmonary arteries (ringlike lucency)

d. the double bronchial wall sign

e. the continuous diaphragm sign

15.Correct positions of tubes and lines are all except

a. Endotracheal tube---3–8 cm above carina

b. Swan–Ganz catheter----superior vena cava

c. Central venous pressure catheter----Superior vena cava

d. Peripherally inserted central catheter line---Superior vena cava

e. Pleural tubes----In pleural space via mid axillary line, 6th to 8th rib spaces.

16.All are true regarding alveolar proteinosis except

a. may simulate the 'bat's wing' appearance of pulmonary oedema

b. 'crazy-paving' pattern

c.bilateral

d.predilection for peripheral lung

e. may be associated with lymphoma and leukaemia

17.All are true regarding pulmonary microlithiasis except

a. the deposition of tiny stones (calcipherites) within alveoli

b. innumerable discrete high-density opacities (resembling grains of sand)

c.bilateral

d. tendency for pulmonary fibrosis and the development of cor pulmonale

e. best demonstrated on an underexposed radiograph

18.All are causes of gross cardiac enlargement except

a. Multiple valve disease

b. Pericardial effusions

c. Dilated cardiomyopathy

d.addison 's disease

e. Arrhythmogenic right ventricular dysplasia

19.The best for unstable patients for assessing left ventricular systolic function

a. CT angiography (CTA)

b.MRA

c.nuclear imaging

d.ECHO

e.angiocardiography

20.The ascending aorta produces a long convexity on the left upper mediastinal contour in

a.TOF

b.UCTGA

c. total superior anomalous pulmonary venous drainage

d. Ebstein's anomaly

e. congenitally corrected transposition (CCTG)

21.All are true except

a. there is usually mirror image branching of the aortic arch in right-sided aortic arch with associated CHD

b. A dilated ascending 'aorta', rising high in the mediastinum is seen typically in persistent arterial truncus or tetralogy of Fallot

c. Rib notching noted in persistent cervical arch (pseudocoarctation)

d. figure of 3 indentation deformity of the left border of the oesophagus is noted in coarctation of aorta

e. figure of 8 noted in total superior anomalous pulmonary venous drainage (Type 1)

22. The study of choice for characterization of the location and extent of regurgitant flow in malfunction of prosthetic valve

a. MRI

b.ECHO

c.MDCT

d.PET

c.Chest x ray

23. The most common cause of congestive heart failure is

a. coronary artery disease

b.valvular heart disease

c.hypertensive heart disease

d.coneginital heart disease

e.cardiomyopathy

24.The most common type of cardiomyopathy

a. congestive cardiomyopathy

b. Hypertrophic cardiomyopathy

c. Restrictive cardiomyopathy

d. Amyloid heart disease

e. Sarcoidosis

25. Features which make 99m Tc to have better imaging characteristics than thallium is /are

a. higher energy

b.less scatter

c.shorter half-life

d.allow use of higher doses

e.easy to produce

26.All are true regarding nuclear cardiac imaging except

a. Resting perfusion abnormalities occur in areas supplied by a very severe (>85%) stenosis

b. stress is often used to increase sensitivity for rate-limiting stenoses

c. adenosine / dipyridamole/dobutamine are used in stress test.

d.current indications for pharmacological perfusion imaging include left bundle branch block and fixed rate pacemaker

e. SPECT may have better specificity than Rubidium-82 for detecting coronary artery disease

27.Radiological features of pulmonary arterial hypertension is/are

a. cardiac enlargement (right atrial and ventricular enlargement)

b.enlargement of the central pulmonary arteries (main pulmonary artery and its branches down to the segmental level)

c.tapering of peripheral arterial branches (vessels beyond segmental level)

d.peripheral pruning

e. all

28.Pulmonary arterial size is said to be enlarged if the transverse diameter of the right descending artery at its midpoint is

a.greater than 16 mm.

b. greater than 17 mm

c. greater than 18 mm

d. greater than 15 mm

e. greater than 19 mm

29..All are true regarding ventilation scintigraphy except

a. ^{133}Xe has longer half-life and lower photon energy (80keV) than ^{81m}Kr

b. ^{133}Xe is cheaper than ^{81m}Kr

c. ^{99m}Tc-DTPA and technegas aerosols can be administered during perfusion imaging

d. aerosol imaging provides a static image of lung ventilation

e. technegas aerosol and ^{81m}Kr better images than diethylene triamine penta-acetate (DTPA)

30.All are true regarding classification of aortic disserction except

a. Distal dissections(Craford) refers to Descending aorta dissection only (distal to left subclavian artery)

b. Type II (DeBakey) refers to Ascending aorta and arch dissection only

c. Type B(Stanford) refers Ascending aorta and arch dissection only

d. Type III IIIa(DeBakey)—limited to thoracic aorta (distal to subclavian artery)dissection

e. Type A(Stanford) refers to aortic dissection proximal to left subclavian artery

31.All are true regarding mediastinal lesions except

a. Most intrathoracic phaeochromocytomas are found in the posterior mediastinum

b. Usually the masses are bilateral and reasonably symmetrical in extramedullary erythropoesis

c. Lymphangiomas are most common in the anterior or superior mediastinum.

d. Mediastinal liposarcomas often occur in the posterior mediastinum

e. mediastinal lipomatosis, is seen in in Cushing's disease

32.The primary imaging investigation used for the diagnosis of aortic dissection

a.chest xray

b.spiral CT

c.MRI

d.PET

e.USG

33.CT angiogram sign is seen in

a.Bronchioloalveolar carcinoma
b.bacterial and lipoid pneumonia
c.pulmonary lymphoma
d.pulmonar infarction and edema
e.all

34.All are true of tuberculosis except

a. lung field often first involved in primary tuberculosis is upper lung
b.apical predominance of lesion is noted in reactivation tuberculosis
c.focal consolidation is a radiographic sign of activity
d.endobronchial spread of infection indicates activity
e.disease activity can be inferred from radiographic resolution of lesions on its empirical treatment

35. Pulmonary hypoplasia is characterized by all except

a. associated asphyxiating thoracic dystrophy

b. a 'bell-shaped' chest and slender ribs

c. evidence of air trapping.

d. may be secondary to diaphragmatic hernia or CCAM resection

e. acquired form overlaps with the Swyer James (MacLeod) syndrome

36.V/Q 'mismatches' means

a.defects on perfusion imaging in regions that are normal on the ventilation study
b.defects on ventilation imaging in regions that are normal on the perfusion study
c.normal on perfusion imaging in regions that are also normal on the ventilation study
d.seen in pulmonary embolism with infarct
e. seen in obstructive airways disease

37.All are true significant aortic disease except

a. critical limb ischaemia belong to Fontaine grade III or IV symptom
b. ABPI (grade IIb 0.5–0.8, grades III–IV <0.5)
c. Angiography is currently the investigation of choice
d. Duplex data acquisition plays significant role in the management
e. MRA is useful

38.All are true regarding aortic occlusive disease except

a. Endovascular techniques are the treatment of choice of chronic aortic occlusive disease
b. Acute aortic occlusive disease is a vascular emergency
c. embolectomy is the treatment of choice in case of irreversible ischemia
d. The key to the diagnosis of acute aortic disease is MRI finding
e. absent Doppler signals indicate irreversible ischemia

39.Potential sources of pulmonary metasatases in paediatric age group are all except
a. Nephroblastoma (Wilms' tumour)

b. Primary bone sarcoma (Ewing or osteosarcoma)

c. Rhabdomyosarcoma

d. Testicular tumour (in the adolescent)

e.ovarian carcinoma

40. Bone involvement in the thorax occur in

a. Neurenteric cyst

b. Neuroblastoma

c. Actinomyces infection

d. Askin tumour

e.all

41.All true regarding interlobular septal thickening except

a.normally a few septa seen

b.commonly seen in interstitial abnormality

c. smooth septal thickening noted in crazy-paving pattern

d.perilobular pattern noted in relation to interlobular septa and the peripheral lobules

e.irregular septal thickening noted in lymphangitic tumour spread

42.Beaded septum sign is noted in

a.pulmonar edema

b.interastitial fibrosis

c.pulmonar haemmorrhage

d.lymphangitic spread

e.all

43.A patient of mitral stenosis undergoes chest x ray which shows cardiac enlargement .All are features of left atrial enlargement except

a.a double right heart border

b.elevation of the left main

bronchus

c.spalying of the carina

d.Hoffman –Rigler sign

e.enlargement of left atrial enlargement

44.The chest x ray of a patient show cardiac enlargement with clearly demarcated cardiac border and no features of any chamber enlargement ,the most likely cause is

a.pericardial effusion

b.constrictive pericarditis

c.dilated cardiomyopathy

d.Mitral stenosis

e.all

45.The gold standard test for pulmonary embolism is

a.CTPA

b.MRA

c.conventional angiography

d.V/Q scan

e.D-dimer

46.All are true regarding conventional pulmonary angiography except

a. The most common nonfatal complications are cardiac arrhythmias and cardiac perforation.

b. pulmonary angiography has a negative sensitivity of up to 99%

c. pulmonary angiography has almost 80% specificity for positive tests

d. only remaining justification at present to perform angiography is before in situ thrombolysis

e. PE may be diagnosed on angiography when an intraluminal filling defect or complete occlusion of an artery is seen.

47.Ancillary signs of pulmonary embolism are all except

a. intravascular filling defect and a 'tram track' appearance

b. small pleural effusions

c.focal infarcts in the costophrenic recesses

d. Enlargement of the bronchial vessels

e. prominent mosaic attenuation pattern

48.Ideal lesion for PCI are all except

a. a short

b.discrete,

c.noncalcified,

d relatively concentric stenosis

e. involve the vessel origin or a branch

49.All are true regarding coronary artery fistula except

a. usually congenital

b. opens most often into the right ventricle

c. The LCA is much more commonly involved than the right

d. associated with cardiac malformations

e.ischemic changes may occur

50.V/Q 'mismatches'means

a.defects on perfusion imaging in regions that are normal on the ventilation study

b.defects on ventilation imaging in regions that are normal on the perfusion study

c.normal on perfusion imaging in regions that are also normal on the ventilation study

d.seen in pulmonary embolism with infarct

e. seen in obstructive airways disease

TEST PAPER 1(ANSWER)

1----e
The two hemidiaphragms are at the same level in some 9% of the population. In a few normal individuals the left hemidiaphragm is up to 1 cm higher than the right. The normal excursion of the diaphragm is usually between 1.5 and 2.5 cm. (G)

2----e
Features that help identify artefacts and skin folds and differentiate from pneumothorax are extension of the 'pneumothorax' line beyond the margin of the chest cavity, laterally located vessels, and an orientation of a line that is inconsistent with the edge of a slightly collapsed lung. In addition, the margin of skin folds tends to be much wider than the normally thin visceral pleural line. (G)

3----c
Pneumothorax in supine positions shows a visible anterior costophrenic recess seen as an oblique line or interface in the hypochondrium; when the recess is manifest as an interface it mimics the adjacent diaphragm ('double diaphragm sign').there is diaphragmatic depression,not diaphragmatic depression. (G)

4---d
Subcarinal lymph node enlargement widens the carinal angle and displaces the azygo-oesophageal line, so that the subcarinal portion of the azygo-oesophageal line, which is normally concave toward the lung, flattens or becomes convex towards the lung, an appearance that may be confused with left atrial enlargement. (Chapter 14,G)

5----e
Posterior mediastinal node enlargement is very unusual. The important diagnostic feature of lymphadenopathy in sarcoidosis is its symmetry .(Chapter 14, G)

6----c
Isolated involvement of the anterior segment of an upper lobe with few exceptions virtually excludes the diagnosis of tuberculosis, although the anterior segment may become involved from contiguous segmental disease. (Chapter 15,G)

7----e
calcification of opacities less common than with primary tuberculosis. (Chapter 15,G)

8----b
Emphysema is characterized by permanent, abnormal enlargement of airspaces distal to the terminal bronchioles. (Chapter 16, G)

9----c
Proteases are normally released in low concentration by phagocytes in the lung. Protease inhibitors,

mainly α_1-protease inhibitor (α_1-antitrypsin), prevent them from causing structural damage to the lung. Imbalance in the protease–antiprotease activity may result from antiprotease deficiency (α_1-antitrypsin deficiency) from excess release of protease stimulated by environmental agents, or from the defective repair of protease-induced damage. (Chapter 16,G)

10----a
Most of pulmonary sarcomas are primay in natue. (Chapter 18, G)

11-----e
Bronchial carcinoids, particularly those located centrally, may calcify and occasionally ossify. Calcification is seen on CT in up to one-third of cases, but is only occasionally visible on chest radiograph. Despite their classification as benign neoplasms, bronchial carcinoids can invade locally and may metastasize to hilar and mediastinal lymph nodes as well as to the brain, liver and bone. (Chapter 18, G)

12----d
Airspace disease, large nodules and pleural effusions are rare in lymphoid interstitial pneumonia (LIP).The cysts in LIP are usually discrete, not found in clusters and are found deep within the lung parenchyma. (Chapter 19, G)

13----e
Clinically significant compression of adjacent airways, arteries and veins is extremely unusual, even though lymph node enlargement is often massive.Stage I—lymphadenopathy, stage II-----lymphadenopathy with parenchymal opacity stage III----parenchymal opacity alone. (Chapter 19, G)

14----b
There is air anterior to pericardium. air on either side of a bronchial wall results in unusually sharp delineation of the wall—the double bronchial wall sign; and air over the diaphragmatic surface leads to the continuous diaphragm sign. .(CHAPTER 20 ,G)

15----b
Swan–Ganz catheter----Right or left pulmonary artery. (CHAPTER 20,G)

16---d
In general, both lungs are involved and airspace opacification is most pronounced in the central lung. on thin-section images a 'crazy-paving' pattern (made up of a striking geographical distribution of ground-glass opacification and thickened interlobular septa) is the characteristic feature of alveolar proteinosis. . (CHAPTER 21,G)

17----e
There is a characteristic radiographic appearance in which innumerable discrete high-density opacities (resembling grains of sand) are seen in both lungs; when profuse there may be a 'white-out' and the tiny stones are then best demonstrated on an overexposed radiograph. . (CHAPTER 21 ,G)

18---d (CHAPTER 22,G)

19---d

Left ventricular systolic function can be assessed with similar accuracy by echocardiography, CT angiography (CTA), MRA, nuclear imaging and angiocardiography. The decision on which to use depends on the need for reproducibility (favouring MRA or nuclear imaging); patient mobility (echocardiography is best for unstable patients where imaging must go to the patient); need for other imaging (selective coronary angiography with angiocardiography); viability (MRI or nuclear imaging); and assessment of valve function (echocardiography). (CHAPTER 22,G)

20---d (CHAPTER 23 ,G)

21----c

There is no rib notching in persistent cervical arch (pseudocoarctation) as there is usually minimal or no stenosis of the aortic lumen. (CHAPTER 23 ,G)

22----b (CHAPTER 24,G)

23----a (CHAPTER 24 ,G)

24-----a (CHAPTER 24 ,G)

25----e (CHAPTER 25 ,G)

26----e

Rubidium-82 may have better specificity than SPECT for detecting coronary artery disease. (CHAPTER 25 ,G)

27----e

In long-standing cases the central pulmonary arteries may develop calcification due to atheroma (a feature not seen in non-

hypertensive pulmonary arteries). (CHAPTER 6 ,G)

28----b (CHAPTER 6,G)

29---c

Tc-DTPA and technegas aerosols cannot be administered during perfusion imaging as both aerosols are labelled with ^{99m}Tc (as used to label the MAA). Aerosol imaging provides a static image of lung ventilation whereas imaging with ^{81m}Kr is more dynamic. Imaging with technegas aerosol has been shown to provide images comparable to those with ^{81m}Kr. (CHAPTER 6,G)

30---c

CLASSIFICATION SYSTEMS FOR AORTIC DISSECTION

	Classification syste		
Site of dissectio	**Crawfo**	**DeBak**	**Stanf**
Both ascendin and descendi aorta	Proxim dissecti	Type I	Type
Ascendi aorta and arch only	Proxim dissecti	Type II	Type
Descend aorta onl (distal to left subclavi artery)	Distal dissecti	Type II IIIa— limited thoraci aorta	Type
		IIIb— extends	

	Classification syste		
Site of dissectio	Crawfo	DeBak	Stanf
		abdomi aorta	

.(CHAPTER 27 ,G)

31---d

Mediastinal liposarcomas are malignant fat-containing tumours. They often occur in the anterior mediastinum where the fat appears heterogeneous on CT. In contradistinction to benign lipomas, they usually contain large areas of soft tissue density material. Lipoblastoma, a benign tumour of childhood, contains fat and soft tissue. (Chapter 14,G)

32----b (CHAPTER 27 ,G)

33----e

CT angiogram sign is said to be present if contrast –enhanced pulmonary vessels appear denser than the surrounding opacified lung (Webb)

34.---a (Webb)

35---c

Unlike Swyer James syndrome, pulmonary hypoplasia shows no evidence of air trapping. .

(CHAPTER 64,G)

36----a (CHAPTER 6 ,G)

37----d

Duplex data acquisition plays very little role in the investigation of significant aortic disease as the aorta is often difficult to visualize and assess. (CHAPTER 27,G)

38----d

The key to the diagnosis of acute aortic disease is the absence of femoral pulses. (CHAPTER 27,G)

39-----e (CHAPTER 64 ,G)

40----e (CHAPTER 64 ,G)

41----e

Irregular septal thickening noted in interstitial fibrosis. Lymphangitic tumour spread shows Smooth or nodular interlobular septal thickening.(Webb).

42----d (Webb)

43-----d

Hoffman-Rigler sign is a sign of left ventricular enlargement.It refers to distance from the posterior aspect of the IVC to the posterior border of the heart horizontally at the level 2cm above the intersection of the diaphragm and the IVC. A distance greater than 1.8 cm indicates left ventricular enlargement.(Sutton)

44----a (Sutton)

45---c (CHAPTER 6 ,G)

46----c

Pulmonary angiography has a negative sensitivity of up to 99% with almost 100% specificity for positive tests. (CHAPTER 6 ,G)

47---a

As in conventional angiography, acute embolism is seen as an

intravascular filling defect.
Contrast medium may be seen to
flow around or adjacent to the clot
(giving a 'tram track' appearance
only if the vessel is in the plane of
the image section). (CHAPTER 6 ,G)

48----e

Ideal lesions for PCI are a short,
discrete, noncalcified, relatively
concentric stenosis that does not
involve the vessel origin or a
branch.(CHAPTER 25,G)

49----c

The fistula opens into the right
heart in 90% of cases, most often
into the right ventricle. The RCA is
much more commonly involved
than the left, although both may be
involved. .(CHAPTER 25 ,G)

50----a (CHAPTER 6 ,G)

TEST PAPER 2

1.Double diaphragm sign is seen in
a. pneumothorax in erect position
b.lamellar effusion
c.basal pleural thickening
d.pneumothorax in supine position
e.diaphragmatic hump

2..Continuous diaphragm sign is seen in
a. Mediastinal haemorrhage
b. Mediastinal emphysema
c. Fibrosing mediastinitis
d.diaphragmatic hernia
e.pericardial effusion

3.Sign almost invariably present with significant tension pneumothorax is
a.ipsilateral mediatinal shift
b.ipsilateral diaphragmatic depression
c. contralateral diaphragmatic depression
d. Double diaphragm sign
e. ipsilateral mediatinal shift

4.All are true regarding pulmonary Kaposi Sarcoma except
a. Unilateral or bilateral pleural fluid (33–50%) and lymphadenopathy (10–30%)
b. poorly defined peribronchovascular nodular opacity (10–20 mm in diameter)
c. bilateral multiple lesions
d. Coarse linear opacities, particularly in the perihilar and lower lungs

e. The lung abnormalities tend to coalesce together like the nodules seen with lymphoma

5.All are true regarding malignant lymphoma except
a.In most cases, the lymphadenopathy is bilateral but asymmetrical.
b.multiple nodal groups are usually involved
c. The posterior mediastinal nodes are infrequently involved
d.Hilar node enlargement is common without accompanying mediastinal node enlargement
e. The anterior mediastinal and paratracheal nodes are the groups most frequently involved

6.All are true regarding Castleman s disease except
a. lymph node hyperplasia of uncertain aetiology
b. the enlarged nodes are usually situated in the middle or posterior mediastinum.
c. can be huge enlargement
d.avascular and so no enhancement
e. The nodes may calcify

7.All are true regarding tuberculoma except
a. seen in post-primary tuberculosis only
b. commonly single nodule of 10-15 mm diameter
c. satellite lesions nearby
d. Calcification common
e. always carry the potential risk of activation and dissemination.

8.All are true regarding emphysema except
a. Centrilobular (centriacinar) emphysema affects mainly the proximal respiratory bronchioles and alveoli in the central part of the acinus
b. Paraseptal emphysema selectively involves the alveoli adjacent to the connective tissues of septa and bronchovascular bundles
c. Panlobular (panacinar) emphysema is characterized by a dilatation of the airspaces of the entire acinus and lobule.
d. Centrilobular (centriacinar) emphysema is the most widespread and severe type of emphysema
e. Irregular (or paracicatricial) emphysema occurs in patients with pulmonary fibrosis

9.All are true regarding emphysema except
a. centrilobular emphysema tends to be most developed in upper parts of the lungs
b. centrilobular emphysema is strongly associated with cigarette smoking
c. panlobular emphysema are often basely predominant
d. emphysema associated with α_1-antitrypsin deficiency is centrilobular (centriacinar) emphysema
e. Irregular (or paracicatricial) emphysema is seen in in pneumoconiosis

10.All are true regarding pulmonary hamartoma except
a. no cavity formation
b.may be part of Carney's triad
c. 90% central
d. Popcorn calcification virtually diagnostic
e. Central fat density on CT

11.All are true regarding tuberculosis except
a. Ill-defined coalesced nodules suggest of active disease
b. poorly marginated linear opacities suggest of active disease
c. cavitary disease suggest of active disease
d. well defined opacities suggest of active disease
e. calcified tuberculous lesions are capable of reactivation.

12.Inflammatory pseudotumour of lung refers to
a. Plasma cell granuloma of the lung
b. Leiomyoma of the lung
c. Sclerosing haemangioma of lung
d. Squamous papillomas of lungs
e. Pulmonary hamartoma

13.All are true regarding lymphadenopathy in sarcoidosis except
a. usually disappears within 6–12 months
b. Recurrence of lymphadenopathy exceedingly rare
c. eggshell calcification of lymph nodes
d. unevenly distributed throughout the mediastinum and hila along the drainage path

e. Nodal enlargement doesnot occur after development of parenchymal opacities.

14.Causes of eggshell nodal calcification are all except

a. Sarcoidosis

b. Silicosis

c. tuberculosis

d. Lymphoma (postirradiation)

e. Amyloidosis

15.Indications of single lung transplantation are all except

a.cystic fibrosis

b. idiopathic pulmonary fibrosis

c.sarcoidosis

d.lymphangioleiomyomatosis

e. emphysema

16.All are true regarding surgical treatmet of emphysema except

a. Bullectomy is considered in patients with a single or several large bullae usually with compression of adjacent lung parenchyma

b.lung transplantation may be used in advanced emphysema

c. LVRS involves the removal of the most severely emphysematous portions of lung in the upper lobes

d. Typically about 50% of each lung is removed in LVRS

e. The NETT overall showed no difference in survival between patients given medical or surgical therapy

17.All are true regarding ejection fraction except

a. the most common index of pump performance

b.EF= (LVEDV-LVESV)/LVEDV

c. Simpson's rule can be used with CT and CMR

d. Simpson's rule is a method for volume or mass calculation

e. Simpson's rule assume that the left ventricle is a prolate ellipse

18.All are true regarding echocardiography

a. the imaging tool used most frequently to evaluate the anatomy and function of the heart

b. the most appropriate method for very sick patients

c. real-time viewing of 3D images not possible

d. Doppler echocardiography display of blood or tissue velocity of heart

e. Pulsed Doppler echocardiography is used to assess localized valve stenosis or regurgitation

19.Features of rib notching in coarctation of aorta are all except

a. the upper margin of the third to eighth ribs

b.usually not seen in children younger than 5 years.)

c. usually bilaterally symmetrical

d. exclusively on the right in aortic coarctation involving the left subclavian artery

e. only on the left in aberrant right subclavian artery arising below the coarctation

20.Atrioventricular endocardial cushion defects is noted in

a. Trisomy chromosome 21

b. Turner's syndrome

c. Noonan's syndrome

d. Holt–Oram syndrome

e. Ellis van Creveld syndrome

21.The most common reason for cardiac transplantation
a. congestive cardiomyopathy
b. Hypertrophic cardiomyopathy
c. Restrictive cardiomyopathy
d. Amyloid heart disease
e. Sarcoidosis

22.All are true regarding imaging of dilated cardiomyopathy except
a.cardiomegaly
b.enlargement of all chambers
c. global hypokinesis
d. delayed enhancement
e. degree of right ventricular dilatation prognostic sign

23.All are true regarding conventional arteriography except
a. Percutaneous femoral arterial catheterization is the usual approach
b. requires at least two shaped catheters
c.Typically 3–10 ml of LOCM is injected for selective coronary angiography
d. requires at least three views for the right coronary artery and five views for the left coronary arteries
e. The overall mortality of coronary angiography is about 0.2% for elective cases

24.All are true regarding mediastinal lesions except
a. Oesophageal perforation is the most frequent cause of acute mediastinitis
b. Fibrosing mediastinitis is usually due to previous infection from histoplasmosis or tuberculosis

c.calcification is seen in fibrosing mediastinitis caused by lymphoma
d. haemorrhage produces an increase in the mediastinal diameter
e.dilatation of esophagus in fibrosing mediastnitis is noted

25.All are true regarding left coronary artery except
a. divides into the left anterior descending (LAD) and circumflex (Cx) coronary arteries
b.LAD give rise to septal and diagonal branches
c. The LAD lies in the anterior interventricular groove on the front of the heart
d. The Cx lies in the left atrioventricular groove
e.In about 25%, the left main coronary has a trifurcation with an intermediate or ramus medianus artery as a branch

26.All are true regarding pulmonary arterial hypertension except
a. the diameter of the main pulmonary artery is greater than that of the adjacent ascending aorta
b. pericardial thickening and effusion
c. vessel distensibility is reduced on MRI
d. calcification due to atheroma seen in non-hypertensive pulmonary arteries
e. mean pulmonary arterial pressure above 30 mmHg during exercise

27.All are true regarding obliterative bronchiolitis except

a. mosaic perfusion on CT

b. vessels have the same calibre in both high and normal attenuation areas

c. Swyer–James or MacLeod syndrome, which is a variant form of postinfectious obliterative bronchiolitis affecting predominantly one lung.

d. CT technique for the assessment of air trapping is based on postexpiratory thin-section images

e. Objective measurement of air trapping can be done using CT densitometry.

28.All are true regarding pulmonary plethora except

a.enlarged central pulmonary arteries

b. visibility of peripheral pulmonary vessels in the outer third of the lung

c.attenuation of peripheral pulmonary vessels

d. most commonly due to a left-to-right shunt in absence of cyanosis

e. A left-to-right shunt of at least 2:1 is required to manifest on x ray

29.All are true regarding CT of aortic dissection except

a. intramural haematoma seen as areas of high attenuation

b. disscction flap visible as a linear track of high attenuation (from intimal calcification) within the aortic lumen on NECT

c. the dissection flap seen as a band of low attenuation on CECT

d. Injection of contrast medium via the left upper limb preferred

e. cobweb sign seen in false lumen

30.Features of false lumen that separate true lumen are all except

a. The false lumen usually tracks around the convexity of the aortic arch

b.false lumen is more often smaller than true lumens

c.The outer wall of the false lumen produces an acute angle at its junction with the dissection flap

d.linear strands of low attenuation within the false lumen (cobweb sign)

e. the true lumen shows continuity with the nondissected aorta.

31.All are true regarding Congenital diaphragmatic hernia except

a. occurs in 1 in 2500 live births.

b. The most common site ---- posterolateral (Bochdalek hernia)

c. Bochdalek hernia involve the left diaphragm in 70% of cases

d. an opacity ,then radiolucencies in affected hemithorax in postnatal period

e. The presence of the stomach in the thorax is usually associated with later herniation and less severe pulmonary hypoplasia

32.All are true regarding Congenital cystic adenomatoid malformation (CAM) except

a. proliferation of bronchiolar structures

b.The prognosis depends on the type rather than the size of lesion

c. CAMs are usually unilobar,

d.usually communicate with the normal tracheobronchial tree

e. receive their blood supply from a normal pulmonary artery and vein

33.Smoking related interstitial lung disease refers to all except
a.Respiratory bronchiolitis
b.RB-ILD
c.desquamative interstitial pneumonitis
d.Langerhans cell histiocytosis
e.constrictive bronchilitis

34.A male patient 35yrs was suffering from of several months of nonproductive cough,low grade fever and shortness of breath with no finger clubbing. PFT of this patient reflect restrictive pattern .The biopsy of lesions shows Masson bodies and patient responded to corticosteroid .HRCT of this patients is expected to show all except
a.patchy bilateral consolidation
b.ground glass opacity/crazy paving
c.subpleural and/or peribronchial distribution more in lower lobe
d.abundant reticular opacity
e. bronchial wall thickening or dilatation in abnormal lung regions

35.All are true of tuberculosis except
a.pleural effusion is more frequent in primary than secondary tuberculosis
b.pleural effusion is always associated with parenchymal lesion in primary tuberculosis

c.organism are uncommonly isolated from pleural fluid in primary tuberculosis
d.pleural thickening and calcification are common finding in advanced tuberculosis
e.pleural abnormalties are usually apical in location

36.All are true of tuberculosis except
a.tree-in-bud appearance reflect endobronchial spread of infection
b. tree-in bud indicates irreversible disease
c. tree-in bud appearance is noted in active TB
d.poorly defined centrinodular nodules or rosettes of nodules indicate active TB
e. centrilobular nodules indicates reversible disease

37.All are true significant aortic disease except
a. critical limb ischaemia belong to Fontaine grade III or IV symptom
b. ABPI (grade IIb 0.5–0.8, grades III–IV <0.5)
c. Angiography is currently the investigation of choice
d. Duplex data acquisition plays significant role in the management
e. MRA is useful

38.All are true regarding aortic occlusive disease except
a. Endovascular techniques are the treatment of choice of chronic aortic occlusive disease
b. Acute aortic occlusive disease is a vascular emergency

c. embolectomy is the treatment of choice in case of irreversible ischemia

d. The key to the diagnosis of acute aortic disease is MRI finding

e. absent Doppler signals indicate irreversible ischemia

39.Potential sources of pulmonary metasatases in paediatric age group are all except

a. Nephroblastoma (Wilms' tumour)

b. Primary bone sarcoma (Ewing or osteosarcoma)

c. Rhabdomyosarcoma

d. Testicular tumour (in the adolescent)

e.ovarian carcinoma

40. Bone involvement in the thorax occur in

a. Neurenteric cyst

b. Neuroblastoma

c. Actinomyces infection

d. Askin tumour

e.all

41.All true regarding interlobular septal thickening except

a.normally a few septa seen

b.commonly seen in interstitial abnormality

c. smooth septal thickening noted in crazy-paving pattern

d.perilobular pattern noted in relation to interlobular septa and the peripheral lobules

e.irregular septal thickening noted in lymphangitic tumour spread

42.Beaded septum sign is noted in

a.pulmonar edema

b.interastitial fibrosis

c.pulmonar haemmorrhage

d.lymphangitic spread

e.all

43.A patient of mitral stenosis undergoes chest x ray which shows cardiac enlargement .All are features of left atrial enlargement except

a.a double right heart border

b.elevation of the left main bronchus

c.spalying of the carina

d.Hoffman –Rigler sign

e.enlargement of left atrial enlargement

44.The chest x ray of a patient show cardiac enlargement with clearly demarcated cardiac border and no features of any chamber enlargement ,the most likely cause is

a.pericardial effusion

b.constrictive pericarditis

c.dilated cardiomyopathy

d.Mitral stenosis

e.all

45. The gold standard test for pulmonary embolism is

a.CTPA

b.MRA

c.conventional angiography

d.V/Q scan

e.D-dimer

46.All are true regarding conventional pulmonary angiography except

a. The most common nonfatal complications are cardiac arrhythmias and cardiac perforation.

b. pulmonary angiography has a negative sensitivity of up to 99%

c. pulmonary angiography has almost 80% specificity for positive tests

d. only remaining justification at present to perform angiography is before in situ thrombolysis

e. PE may be diagnosed on angiography when an intraluminal filling defect or complete occlusion of an artery is seen.

47.Ancillary signs of pulmonary embolism are all except

a. intravascular filling defect and a 'tram track' appearance

b. small pleural effusions

c.focal infarcts in the costophrenic recesses

d. Enlargement of the bronchial vessels

e. prominent mosaic attenuation pattern

48.Ideal lesion for PCI are all except

a. a short

b.discrete,

c.noncalcified,

d relatively concentric stenosis

e. involve the vessel origin or a branch

49.All are true regarding coronary artery fistula except

a. usually congenital

b. opens most often into the right ventricle

c. The LCA is much more commonly involved than the right

d. associated with other cardiac malformations (e.g. pulmonary atresia, patent ductus arteriosus)

e.ischemic changes may occur

50.Correct matching of lung disease and pathology are all except

a. Flock worker's lung--- Lymphocytic bronchiolitis

b. Flavour worker's lung-- Obliterative bronchiolitis

c. Berylliosis----caseating granulomas

d. Hard metal pneumoconiosis-- Giant cell interstitial pneumonia

e.Sarcoidosis --- Noncaseating granulomas

TEST PAPER 2(ANSWER)

1---d (G)

2----b

In Mediastinal emphysema ,air may track extraserosally on either side of the diaphragm, which is occaisionally seen as a continuous line of transradiancy known as the 'continuous diaphragm sign'. (Chapter 14,G)

3----b

Moderate or gross mediastinal shift should be taken as indicating tension, particularly if the ipsilateral hemidiaphragm is depressed. Depreesed ipsilateral hemidiaphragm is the more reliable and is almost invariably present with significant tension pneumothorax. **(G)**

4---e

The lung abnormalities tend to coalesce together unlike the nodules seen with lymphoma. Rapid progression from a poorly-defined nodular pattern to one of airspace consolidation has usually been seen in patients with haemoptysis, and probably represents haemorrhage into the lung. (Chapter 15,G)

5---d

Hilar node enlargement is rare without accompanying mediastinal node enlargement, particularly in Hodgkin's disease. The paracardiac nodes are rarely involved but become important as sites of recurrent disease because they may not be included in the initial radiation therapy fields. (Chapter 14, G)

6----d

Castleman's disease is a specific type of lymph node hyperplasia of uncertain aetiology which can cause substantial lymph node enlargement in many sites in the body. The lymph node mass may be very vascular and may show striking contrast enhancement on both CT and MRI. (Chapter 14,G)

7----a

A tuberculoma may occur in the setting of primary or post-primary tuberculosis and probably represents localized parenchymal disease that alternately activates and heals. (Chapter 15, G)

8---d

Panlobular (panacinar) emphysema is the most widespread and severe type of emphysema. (Chapter 16,G)

9---d

Panlobular emphysema is the type of emphysema that occurs in α_1-antitrypsin deficiency and in familial cases. (Chapter 16,G)

10----c

The distribution of pulmonary hamartomas is opposite to that seen with bronchial carcinoid: 90% are peripheral and present as a solitary pulmonary nodule, while the remaining 10% arise within a major bronchus.

A triad of pulmonary chondroma(s) (often multiple), gastric epithelioid leiomyosarcoma (leiomyoblastoma) and functioning extra-adrenal paragangliomas are known as Carney's triad (Chapter 18,G)

11---d

Ill-defined coalesced nodules, poorly marginated linear opacities, and especially cavitary disease in the appropriate segments are suspicious for active disease, whereas well defined opacities are not. Exceptions occur, however, and clinical findings are necessary for the diagnosis. (Chapter 15,G)

12---a

Plasma cell granuloma of the lung (inflammatory pseudotumour) is the name given to a lesion that is presumed to be reactive inflammatory granulomatous tissue. (Chapter 18,G)

13----d

Lymph node calcification is seen on the radiograph in 5% or less of patients with sarcoidosis, it may be evident on CT in up to 40% of patients with long-standing disease. The affected lymph nodes are usually small in volume and evenly distributed throughout the mediastinum and hila (very different from calcified nodes due to tuberculous infection which usually follow a drainage path). About 40% of patients presenting with nodal enlargement will develop parenchymal opacities, usually within a year, and of these about one-third will go on to have persistent (fibrotic) shadowing. (Chapter 19, G)

14----c

Causes of eggshell nodal calcification are sarcoidosis. silicosis, lymphoma (postirradiation),amyloidosis, histoplasmosis, blastomycosis. (Chapter 19,G)

15---a

Bilateral sequential lung transplantation is performed for suppurative lung diseases, such as cystic fibrosis and bronchiectasis and also for severe pulmonary hypertension. (CHAPTER 20,G)

16---d

LVRS involves the removal of the most severely emphysematous portions of lung in the upper lobes. Typically about 30% of each lung is removed using either a median sternotomy or a video-assisted thoracoscopic technique. . (CHAPTER 20 ,G)]

17----e

Simpson's rule is a method for volume or mass calculation based on dividing the ventricular volume into a series of slices equidistant along the long axis of the ventricle. It makes no assumption about the shape of the ventricle.(CHAPTER 22 ,G)

18----c

Through computer reconstruction of 2D images, 3D echocardiograms have become possible. New, faster techniques are making real-time viewing of 3D images possible. .(CHAPTER 22 .G)

19----a

Rib notching of the lower margin of the third to eighth ribs is noted in aortic coarctation due to the enlarged, tortuous intercostal arteries supplying blood to (instead of conducting blood from) the descending aorta. (CHAPTER 23,G)

20---a (CHAPTER 23 ,G)

21----a (CHAPTER 24,G)

22----d

Regional wall thinning and delayed enhancement are seen in ischemic cardiomyopathy. Severe right ventricular dilatation is a poor prognostic sign. A normal right ventricle should raise suspicions of global left ventricular impairment due to multiple infarctions from ischaemic heart disease. (CHAPTER 24 ,G)

23---b

Percutaneous femoral arterial catheterization is the usual approach and requires at least three shaped catheters, one for each coronary artery, and one for the left ventricle (usually a pigtail configuration). (CHAPTER 25 .G)

24--- c

Calcification of hilar or mediastinal lymphnodes is noted in histoplasmosis/tuberculosis, which is an important feature for differentiating fibrosing mediastinitis from other infiltrative disorders of the mediastinum, such as lymphoma and metastatic carcinoma. (Chapter 14, G)

25----e

In about 10% the left main coronary has a trifurcation with an intermediate or ramus medianus artery, arising between the LAD and Cx coronary arteries . This vessel is effectively a diagonal branch serving the lateral aspect of the left ventricle. (CHAPTER 25.G)

26----d (CHAPTER 6 ,G)

.27---b

The vessels within areas of decreased attenuation in obliterative bronchiolitis on thin-section CT may be of markedly reduced calibre, they are not distorted as in emphysema. The lung areas of decreased attenuation related to decreased perfusion can be patchy or widespread. They are poorly defined or sharply demarcated, giving a geographical outline, and represent a collection of affected secondary pulmonary lobules. Redistribution of blood flow to the normally ventilated areas causes increased attenuation of lung parenchyma in these areas. The patchwork of abnormal areas of low attenuation and normal lung or less diseased areas, appearing normal in attenuation or hyperattenuated, gives the appearance of mosaic attenuation. The vessels in the abnormal hypoattenuated areas are reduced in calibre, whereas the vessels in normal areas are increased in size; the resulting pattern is called mosaic perfusion. The difference in vessel size between low and high attenuation areas allows the mosaic perfusion pattern to be distinguished from mosaic attenuation due to an infiltrative lung disease with patchy distribution, in which the vessels have the same calibre in both high and normal attenuation areas. (Chapter 16, G)

28----c

Radiologically, the central pulmonary arteries enlarge in

pulmonary plethora In addition, peripheral pulmonary vessels become visible in the outer third of the lung—a sign known as 'pulmonary plethora' (unlike in PAH where there is enlargement of central arteries with peripheral arterial pruning). (CHAPTER 6 ,G)

29----d
Injection of contrast medium via the left upper limb should be avoided as the very high attenuation from contrast medium within the left brachiocephalic vein can produce streak artefact across the aortic arch, potentially causing diagnostic difficulty . (CHAPTER 27 ,G)

30---b
The false lumen usually tracks around the convexity of the aortic arch and is more often than not the larger of the two lumens. Occasionally, linear strands of low attenuation may be seen within the false lumen (cobweb sign). These represent residual strands of media incompletely sheared away at the time of dissection. (CHAPTER 27 ,G)

31---e
The presence of the stomach in the thorax is usually associated with earlier herniation and mpr severe pulmonary hypoplasia. **(CHAPTER 64 .G)**

32----b
The prognosis depends on the size rather than the type of lesion. **(CHAPTER 64 .G)**

33---e (Webb)

34----d
The case is of BOOP /Cryptogenic organizing pneumonia .Presence of consolidation and paucity of reticular opacity differentiate it from IPF.(Webb)

35----b
Pleural effusion is unassociated with ovious parenchymal lesion in primary tuberculosis

36--- b
Tree-in bud indicates reversible disease (Webb)

37----d
Duplex data acquisition plays very little role in the investigation of significant aortic disease as the aorta is often difficult to visualize and assess. (CHAPTER 27 ,G)

38----d
The key to the diagnosis of acute aortic disease is the absence of femoral pulses. (CHAPTER 27.G)

39----e (CHAPTER 64 .G)

40---e (CHAPTER 64 ,G)

41----e
Irregular septal thickening noted in interstitial fibrosis. Lymphangitic tumour spread shows Smooth or nodular interlobular septal thickening.(Webb).

42----d (Webb)

43----d
Hoffman-Rigler sign is a sign of left ventricular enlargement.It refers to distance from the posterior aspect of the IVC to the posterior border of the heart horizontally at the level 2cm above the

intersection of the diaphragm and the IVC. A distance greater than 1.8 cm indicates left ventricular enlargement.(Sutton)

44----a (Sutton)

45---c (CHAPTER 6 ,G)

46----c

Pulmonary angiography has a negative sensitivity of up to 99% with almost 100% specificity for positive tests. (CHAPTER 6 ,G)

47----a

As in conventional angiography, acute embolism is seen as an intravascular filling defect. Contrast medium may be seen to flow around or adjacent to the clot (giving a 'tram track' appearance only if the vessel is in the plane of the image section). (CHAPTER 6,G)

48---e

Ideal lesions for PCI are a short, discrete, noncalcified, relatively concentric stenosis that does not involve the vessel origin or a branch.(CHAPTER 25 .G)

49----c

The fistula opens into the right heart in 90% of cases, most often into the right ventricle. The RCA is much more commonly involved than the left, although both may be involved. .(CHAPTER 25.G)

50----c

Berylliosis shows noncaseating granulomas. (Chapter 19, G)

TEST PAPER 3

1.An old white female of 35 yrs presented with renal disease , paranasal sinus pain, bloody nasal discharge ,cough and hemoptysis .Lab study reveals elevated ESR,mildly elevated rheumatoid factor and a positive antiproteinase -3 ANCA.All would be finding on CT scan of this patient except
a.multiple ,bilateral lesions
b.nodular lesions
c.cavitatory lesions
d.peripheral and pleural based lesions
e.the CT Halo sign

2. An old female patient of 60 yrs after undergoing total hip replacement developed unexplained breathlessness and chest pain and tachypnea .The patient showed hypoxemia (decreased arterial PO_2) and an increased alveolar-arterial O_2 tension gradient.The d-dimer is abnormally elevated.Pulmonary CT angio is most likely to reveal
a.Tram track appearance
b.signet ring appearance
c.hyperdynamic circulation
d.rapid run-off
e.feeding vessel

3.All are true of neonatal pulmonary infection except
a. Pleural effusions frequently occur in group B streptococcal infection
b. Pneumatocele formation is common in the neonate
c.pneumatocele may be seen in association with *E. coli ,Haemophilus influenzae, Staph. aureus*
d. Chlamydial infection does not produce pulmonary disease until 4–6 weeks
e. overinflation with marked bilateral symmetric interstitial changes seen in Chlamydial infection

4.The most common cause of an isolated pleural effusion in neonate is
a. Chylothorax
b. Haemophilus influenza
c. Staph. Aureus
d.E.coli
e.meconeum aspiration

5.All are true regarding traumatic aortic injury except
a. a linear filling defect in dissection on angiography
b. usually an obtuse margin at the junction of the abnormal and normal aortic wall in pseudoaneurysm
c. Transoesophageal echocardiography (TOE) has a sensitivity of 91% and specificity of 98% for demonstration of isthmic aortic injuries

d. direct signs of aortic trauma on CT are intramural haematoma and contrast extravasation

e. endovascular repair of TAI ideally requires at least 15 mm of aorta proximal to the injury

6.All are true regarding aortic dissection except

a. Aortic dissection ---the most common non-traumatic acute aortic emergency

b. related to advancing age and hypertension

c. cleavage plane between the outer two-thirds and inner one-third of media

d. intramural haematoma and penetrating atherosclerotic ulcer --- supposed precursors of dissection

e. Intramural haematoma distinguished from mural thrombus with cross-sectional imaging

7. Pulmonary arterial hypertension (PAH) refers to an elevation in mean pulmonary arterial pressure above

a.30 mmHg during exercise (and 25 mmHg at rest)

b. 25 mmHg during exercise (and 20 mmHg at rest).

c. 35 mmHg during exercise (and 30 mmHg at rest)

d. 20 mmHg during exercise (and 15 mmHg at rest)

e. 25 mmHg during exercise (and 30 mmHg at rest)

8.Cause of pulmonary arterial hypertention is/are

a. Chronic lung disease

b. Pulmonary embolic disease

c. Pulmonary venous hypertension

d. left-to-right or bidirectional shunts

e.All

9.First-line technique for evaluating myocardial perfusion, viability and function is

a.Echo

b. Nuclear cardiac imaging

c.CMR

d.MDCT

e.X ray

10.All are myocardial perfusion agents except

a. SestaMIBI (^{99m}Tc-methoxyisobutyl-isonitrile)

b.Tetrofosmin

c.Teboroxime

d. Thallium

e.Strontium

11.Mechanical Valves in common use is

a. the Bjork–Shiley,Omniscience, and Medtronic–Hall --- Eccentric monocuspid disc valve

b. St Jude ,the Carbomedics and Sorin bicarbon valves---- Bileaflet disc valve

c. the Beall and Starr–Edwards 6500 series.----   Central caged disc occluder valve

d. the Starr–Edwards, Harken, Smelloff–Cutter---- Central ball occluder valve

e. Carpentier–Edwards ,the Hancock and the Ionescu–Shiley ----bioprostheses

12.Which is used in cardiac valvuloplasty

a.Duran ring

b.Carpentier–Edwards ring

c. Hancock ring

d. St Jude

e. Carbomedics

 13.Figure of 8 is noted in

a.TOF

b.UCTGA

c. total superior anomalous pulmonary venous drainage(Type 1)

d. Ebstein's anomaly

e. Uhl's disease

14.A vascular pedicle which is narrow in the frontal view and wide on the lateral radiograph is seen in

a.TOF

b.UCTGA

c. total superior anomalous pulmonary venous drainage

d. Ebstein's anomaly

e. Uhl's disease

15.The most frequently used method for assessing left ventricular dimensions and function

a. echocardiography

b.CT

c.MRI

d.PET –CT

e.Chest xray

16.Most common cause of left ventricular renlargement

a. Cardiomyopathy

b. Mitral regurgitation

c. Myocardial ischaemia

d. Aortopulmonary window

e. systemic hypertension

17.All are true regarding COP except

a. 'reverse halo' sign

b. Type II linear opacities not related to airways

c. perilobular pattern

d. Type I opacities intimately related to bronchi and extend radially towards the pleura

e. Type II linear opacities sub-pleural and perpendicular to pleural surface

18.Chest radiographic appearance of TOF are all except

a. right ventricular heart silhouette

b.boot-shaped heart

c. pulmonary oligaemia

d. concave pulmonary artery segment

e. large hila

19.All are true regarding eosinophilic lung disease except

a. transient and fleeting radiographic infiltrates in simple pulmonary eosinophilia (Löffler's syndrome)

b. may be spontaneous resolution of acute eosinophilic pneumonia

c. consolidation typically in the mid and lower zones in chronic eosinophilic pneumonia

d. 'photographic negative of pulmonary oedema' in chronic eosinophilic pneumonia

e. the opacities peripheral and s parallel the chest wall in chronic eosinophilic pneumonia

20. Acute respiratory distress syndrome is characterized by all except

a. exudative phase, proliferative phase , a fibrotic phase

b. normal pulmonary capillary wedge pressure

c. pleural effusion very common

d. ratio of arterial to inspired

fraction of oxygen of less than 300 mmHg

e. a more peripheral distribution of airspace opacities than that of cardiogenic pulmonary oedema

21.All are true regarding typical CT finding of ARDS

a.more frequent in cases of extrapulmonary causes

b. consolidation in the dependent, posterior parts of the lung

c. usually gradual reduction in density from dependant to nondependent areas

d. normal lung in the most anterior portion of the chest

e. Cystic spaces

22.All are true regarding RB–ILD except

a. patchy ground-glass opacification

b. well- defined high attenuation centrilobular nodules

c. upper lobe centrilobular emphysema

d. areas of air trapping

e. strong association with cigarette smoking

23. Smoking related-interstitial lung disease (SR-ILD) include all except

a. DIP

b. RB–ILD

c.LCH .

d. Cryptogenic organizing pneumonia

e. interstitial fibrosis

24.All are true regarding invasion by bronchogenic tumour except

a. phrenic nerve paralysis may be

evidence of mediastinal invasion

b. MRI offer significant advantages over CT for the routine diagnosis of mediastinal invasion

c. The presence of chest wall invasion alone does not preclude surgical resection

d. MRI is regarded as the optimal modality for demonstrating the extent of superior sulcus tumours

e. ^{99m}Tc radionuclide skeletal scintigraphy is a sensitive technique to assess bone invasion

25.All are true regarding intrathoracic lymph nodes metastases except

a.skip metastases to mediastinal nodes in the absence of hilar nodes is seen in 53% of cases

b.mediastinal nodes with a short axis diameter more than than 10 mm should usually be considered enlarged.

c.Fused PET–CT imaging is more accurate than PET or CT alone in staging patients with non-small cell lung cancer .

d. Mediastinoscopy and mediastinotomy remain the most widely employed techniques for mediastinal lymph node sampling

e. the MRI signal within nodes is not a useful predictor of involvement of nodes

26.All are true regarding chronic changes of ABPA except

a. central location of bronchectasis

b. cystic or varicose bronchectasis more likely

c. High attenuation within the plugs

d. upper lobar shrinkage
e. lower lobe predilection of bronchectasis

27. All are true regarding bronchiectasis except

a. internal bronchial diameter greater than that of the adjacent pulmonary artery (signet ring sign)
b. The combination of bronchiectasis, sinusitis and situs inversus is termed Kartagener's syndrome
c. bilateral bronchiectasis with a upper lobe predominance is noted in Dyskinetic cilia syndrome
d. Cylindrical bronchiectasis is the most common type of bronchectasis seen in Dyskinetic cilia syndrome
e. Bronchoceles is seen in ABPA

28. All are true regarding tuberculous miliary lesions except

a. classically a manifestation of primary disease
b. Multiple small (1–2 mm) discrete nodules
c. Calcification within miliary nodules very common
d. scattered evenly throughout both lung field
e. no residual changes after therapy

29. All are true regarding primary tuberculosis except

a. the primary pneumonia usually resolves completely
b. segmental or lobar collapse in primary tuberculosis commonly in the posterior segment of the right upper lobe and the middle lobe

c. a Ghon lesion or focus refers to a residual well defined rounded or irregular (linear) opacity, with or without calcification
d. Nodal calcification may occur in the ipsilateral hilum or mediastinum and is heterogeneous and irregular
e. When a Ghon lesion and ipsilateral lymph node calcification are seen together the combination is termed a Ranke complex

30. All are likely causes of mediastinal or hilar lymph nodes greater than 2cm in short axis in diameter except

a. pneumoconiosis
b. metastatic carcinoma
c. malignant lymphoma
d. sarcoidosis
e. tuberculosis

31. All are likely causes of mediastinal or hilar lymph nodes greater than 2cm in short axis in diameter except

a. pneumoconiosis
b. metastatic carcinoma
c. malignant lymphoma
d. sarcoidosis
e. tuberculosis

32. The curving of pulmonary vessels or bronchi into the edge of the lesion which is abutting the pleural surface is known as

a. the comet-tail sign
b. the Head-Cheese sign
c. halo sign
d. crazy-paving
e. Romana sign

33. The most common

manifestation and the most characteristic radiographic feature of asbestos exposure is

a.parietal pleural plaques
b.round atelectasis
c.dotlike opacities
d.parenchymal bands
e.subpleural lines

34.All are true regarding cardiac myxoma except

a. 75% arises in the left atrium
b.solitary
c.pedunculated or polypoid
d.more in women
e. 85% of cases attached to anterior wall

35.All are true of familial cardiac myxoma except

a. fewer than 10% of all myxomas
b. tend to present in older age (median age 50 years)
c. more likely be to multiple
d. atypical locations
e.develop recurrent tumours

36 Which is used in CABG surgery ?

a. left internal mammary artery
b. the right internal mammary artery
c. gastro-epiploic artery
d. saphenous vein
e.all

37.All are true regarding Left ventricular aneurysm except

a. aneurysms are akinetic
b. False aneurysm fills and empties slowly with contrast medium
c. no myocardium in the wall of the false aneurysm
d. enhancement on DE-MRI in false aneurysm

e. reversal of curvature at the 'neck' must for diagnosis

38.A normal V/Q study has been shown to have a negative predictive value of

a.100%
b. 80%
c. 70%
d. 60%
e. 50%

39.A patient suffering from tuberculosis was suffering from increasing dyspnea and so requested for chest xary. The finding which favour constrictive pericarditis is

a.pericardial calcification in anterior aspect
b. pericardial calcification in lateral aspect
c pericardial calcification in posterior aspect
d. pericardial calcification in atrioventricular groove
e.straighetning of right heart border

40.All are true regarding asbestos-related disease (pleural plaque) except

a. involve the visceral pleural almost exclusively
b.distributed along the posterolateral chest wall between the 7th and 10th ribs,
c.distributed along lateral chest wall between the 6th and 9th ribs,
d.distributed along the dome of the diaphragm
e.distributed along the mediastinal pleura

41.All are true regarding round

atelectasis /folded lung except

a. a form of parenchymal collapse

b. most commonly in the peripheral lung in the dorsal regions of the upper lobes

c. comet tail sign

d. Volume loss of the affected lobe invariably present

e. usually rounded or oval shape

42.Early CT changes indicative of asbestosis are all except

a the presence of subpleural curvilinear lines and dots

b. pleural-based nodular irregularities

c. parenchymal bands and

d.septal lines

e. honeycombing

43.CT may be reliably used to detect emboli in up to

a. fourth-order vessels

b. third -order vessels

c.second –order vessels

d.sixth- order order vessels

e.fifth -order vessels

44.All are technical considerations in doing CTPA except

a. whole lung may be examined during a single breath-hold in almost all patients in MDCT

b. an iodine concentration of 350 mg ml⁻ or more injected at a rate of 4–5 ml s⁻ and a volume of 120–140 ml is recommended

c. streak artefact may be seen in case of high iodine concentration

d. superior vena cava thrombosis and persistent intracardiac shunts reduce adequacy of opacification.

e. middle lobe arteries which often run tangential to the plane of a conventional transverse image

45.All are true regarding DVT except

a. 90% of PEs result from DVT

b. contrast medium studies is the 'gold standard'study

c. US the first choice of investigation for suspected DVT in patients with nondiagnostic PE investigations

d. CT venography need additional contrast after doing CTPA

e. MRI allows distinction between acute and chronic DVT

46.The most common cyanotic congenital heart defect

a. tetralogy of Fallot

b. uncorrected transposition of great arteries (UTGA).

c. common atria and common ventricles

d. PDA

e. persistent truncus arteriosus

47.All are true regarding myocardial stunning except

a. refers to prolonged but temporary ventricular dysfunction

b. follows a period of ischaemia

c. myocardium is viable

d. retains contrast on DE-MRI

e. recovery of left ventricular function during extended pharmacological stress testing

48.All are true of TOF except

a. right ventricular outflow (RVOT) obstruction

b. a subaortic VSD

c. aortic override

d. right ventricular hypertrophy

e. malalignment of the interartrial septum

49. All are true regarding Bland–Garland–White syndrome except
a. left coronary artery arising from the pulmonary artery
b. right coronary artery arising from the pulmonary artery
c. collateral retrograde flow from the RCA
d. chest x-ray simulated dilated cardiomyopathy
e. The diagnosis is usually obvious on aortography

50. The imaging modality of choice for initial diagnosis and assessment
a. Trans-thoracic echocardiography
b. chest x ray
c. MDCT
d. MRI
e. MRA

TEST PAPER 3(ANSWER)

1----e

This is a case of Wegener's granulomatosis which shows the feeding vessel sign (nodule or focal opacity that demonstrates a vessel leading to it) The CT halo sign consists of a round pulmonary mass or nodule with a surrounding halo of intermediate CT attenuation,noted in invasive pulmonary aspergillosis (Hagga)

2----a

As in conventional angiography, acute embolism is seen as an intravascular filling defect.
Contrast medium may be seen to flow around or adjacent to the clot (giving a 'tram track' appearance only if the vessel is in the plane of the image section).(Grainger)

3-----b

Pneumatocele formation is uncommon in the neonate .
(CHAPTER 64,G)

4----a (CHAPTER 64,G)

5---b

In pseudoaneurysm, discontinuity or asymmetry/irregularity of the aortic contour may be seen on angiography . There is usually an acute margin at the junction of the abnormal and normal aortic wall, differentiating a pseudoaneurysm from a ductus diverticulum, which classically has a smooth symmetrical contour and obtuse margins with the 'normal' aorta. (CHAPTER 27 ,G)

6----c

The classic dissection is initiated by an intimal tear, which allows blood to penetrate into and split the medial layer. A cleavage plane is produced between the inner two-thirds and outer one-third of media.(CHAPTER 27,G)

7---a (CHAPTER 6,G)

8---e (CHAPTER 6 ,G)

9----b (CHAPTER 25,G)

10---e (CHAPTER 25 ,G)

11---b (CHAPTER 24 ,G)

12---a (CHAPTER 24 ,G

13----c (CHAPTER 23 ,G)

14----b (CHAPTER 23 ,G)

15----e

The feature that best characterizes left ventricular morphology is fibrous continuity of the entry atrioventricular valve and the exit semilunar valve, due to the lack of any conus or infundibulum. (CHAPTER 22 ,G)

16----c (CHAPTER 22 ,G)

17---e

Type II linear opacities tend to be parallel to the pleural surface but like Type I changes are frequently associated with multifocal airspace consolidation. (CHAPTER 21 ,G)

18---e Small hila is noted in TOF. (CHAPTER 23,G)

19---c

The plain radiographic abnormalities in chronic eosinophilic pneumonia may be characteristic: patchy, nonsegmental areas of consolidation are typical in the mid and upper zones. A distinctive feature is that the opacities are peripheral and seem to parallel the chest wall, a finding that has been called the 'photographic negative of pulmonary oedema'. (CHAPTER 21 ,G)

20----c
Pleural effusions are seldom seen on the supine radiographs obtained on such patients. (CHAPTER 20 ,G)

21----e
Cystic spaces were a feature of the atypical appearance of ARDS. The most common abnormality in the survivors of ARDS is a reticular pattern (indicating fibrosis) and this had a striking anterior distribution .(CHAPTER 20 ,G)

22----b
On HRCT, the features of RB–ILD include areas of patchy ground-glass opacification (resulting from macrophage accumulation within alveolar spaces and alveolar ducts) and poorly defined low attenuation centrilobular nodules. (Chapter 19, G)

23----d
Smoking related-interstitial lung disease (SR-ILD) has been proposed to encompass DIP, RB–ILD, LCH and interstitial fibrosis. (Chapter 19, G)

24----b
MRI does not appear to offer any advantages over CT for the routine diagnosis of mediastinal invasion, its role being limited to problem solving in specific cases. (Chapter 18, G)

25----a
Lung cancers normally spread to ipsilateral hilar nodes, then ipsilateral mediastinal, contralateral mediastinal and supraclavicular nodes. Though nodal spread is most often sequential, skip metastases to mediastinal nodes in the absence of hilar nodes is seen in 33% of cases. (Chapter 18, G)

26----e
There is upper lobe predilection of bronchectasis in ABPA. (Chapter 16, G)

27----c
Bilateral bronchiectasis with a basal (lower or middle lobe) predominance is noted in Dyskinetic cilia syndrome. (Chapter 16,G

28----c
Calcification within miliary nodules is rare or nonexistent. (Chapter 15, G)

29----b
Nodal pressure and bronchial erosion in primary tuberculosis may cause segmental or lobar collapse; commonly in the anterior segment of the right upper lobe and the middle lobe. (Chapter 15, G)

30---a

When mediastinal or hilar nodes are greater than 2 cm in their short axis diameter, the enlargement is likely to be due to metastatic carcinoma, malignant lymphoma, sarcoidosis, tuberculosis, or fungal infection. With lesser degrees of enlargement the differential diagnosis broadens to include lymph node hyperplasia and pneumoconiosis. Widespread moderate mediastinal lymph node enlargement is a frequent accompaniment of chronic diffuse lung disease and bronchiectasis. (Chapter 14, G)

31---a

When mediastinal or hilar nodes are greater than 2 cm in their short axis diameter, the enlargement is likely to be due to metastatic carcinoma, malignant lymphoma, sarcoidosis, tuberculosis, or fungal infection. With lesser degrees of enlargement the differential diagnosis broadens to include lymph node hyperplasia and pneumoconiosis. Widespread moderate mediastinal lymph node enlargement is a frequent accompaniment of chronic diffuse lung disease and bronchiectasis. (Chapter 14, G)

32----a (Webb)

33----a (Webb)

34----e

85% of cases of cardiac myxoma is characteristically attached to the interatrial septum near the fossa ovalis. (CHAPTER 24 ,G)

35---b

Familial myxomas constitute fewer than 10% of all myxomas, tend to present earlier (median age 20 years) and have associated dermatological and endocrine abnormalities (Carney complex). (CHAPTER 24 ,G)

36----e (CHAPTER 25 ,G)

37----d

There is no myocardium in the wall of the false aneurysm, and unlike a true aneurysm there is no enhancement on DE-MRI. False aneurysms have a tendency to rupture and should be excised. (CHAPTER 25 ,G)

38----a (CHAPTER 6 ,G)

39----c

Calcification doesnot occur at the back of the heart as fluid cannot collect around the insertion

40---a

Pleural plaque involve the parietal pleural almost exclusively. Calcification is reported in 10–15% of cases. (Chapter 19, G)

41----b

The round pneumonia shows crowding of bronchi and blood vessels that extend from the border of the mass to the hilum ('comet tail' sign). (Chapter 19, G)

42----b (Chapter 19, G)

43----a (CHAPTER 6 ,G)

44---b

An iodine concentration of 120-250 mg ml$^-$ injected at a rate of 4–5 ml s$^-$ and a volume of 120–140 ml is recommended. Experience has shown that high concentration contrast media (350 mg ml⁻ of iodine or greater) are associated with significant streak artefact (e.g. in the superior vena cava), which can obscure accurate assessment of embolism. (CHAPTER 6 ,G)

45----d
CT should be performed with a suitable delay (in the order of 3 min) after CTPA, thus obviating the need for further contrast medium. (CHAPTER 6,G)

46----a
Tetralogy of Fallot is the most common cyanotic congenital heart defect with an incidence of approximately 420 per million live births. The prevalence of Eisenmenger syndrome has declined as diagnosis and surgical closure of shunts has greatly improved. (CHAPTER 23.G)

47.---d
In stunning of myocardium ,there is abnormal ventricular function but the myocardium is viable, has contractile reserve, and can regain normal function with revascularization. Stunning can be seen after relief of ischaemia by thrombolysis, PCI, coronary bypass grafting, reversal of vasospasm, or after exercise. Stunning can be identified by recovery of left ventricular function during extended pharmacological stress testing with imaging by echocardiography, radionuclide imaging, or cine-MRA(Edelman)

48----e
TOF is caused by malalignment of the infundibular septum. (CHAPTER 23 ,G)

49----c
In Bland–Garland–White syndrome ,left coronary artery arises from the pulmonary artery with collateral retrograde flow from the RCA. .(CHAPTER 25 ,G)

50----a (CHAPTER 23 ,G)

TEST PAPER 4

1.40 yrs old male suffered RTA and brought to emergency within two hrs.The immediate chest x ray of the patients showed nonsegmental consolidation adjacent to the ribs and the subsequent CT scan showed the irregular hyperdense lesions with subpleural predominance which cleared within a week. There is no pneumatocele What is the most likely diagnosis?

a. acute respiratory distress syndrome

b. fat embolism

c. Pulmonary laceration

d. Pulmonary contusion

e. Lung torsion

2.Elderly female, under treatment of invasice breast cancer was admitted for investigation of her increasing cough and difficulty in breathing .Her chest x ray showed fine reticulonodular shadowing and thickened septal lines and subpleural oedema with right sided pleural effusion . High-resolution CT showed nonuniform, nodular, thickening of the interlobular septa and irregular thickening of the bronchovascular bundles in the central portions of the both lungs . Many of the acini subtended by thickened interlobular septa were normally aerated. Thers is no hilar lymph node enlargement.The most likely cause of her symptom is

a.PCP

b.drug sensitivity

c.metastases

d.lymphangitis carcinomatosis

e.invasive aspergillosis

3.All are true regarding lung development except

a. primitive lung buds are present by the sixth week

b. True alveolar development starts from approximately 26 weeks gestation

c. True alveolar development stops within week of birth

d. Surfactant is produced from about 24 weeks gestation

e. The lamellar bodies appear at around 22 weeks gestation

4.Surfactant is produced

a.within the endoplasmic reticulum of type 2 pneumocytes

b. within the golgi body of type 2 pneumocytes

c. within the endoplasmic reticulum of type 1 pneumocytes

d. within the golgi body of type 1 pneumocytes

e. within the mitochondria of type 2 pneumocytes

5.Bronchiectasis may be seen in

all except

a.Kartagener syndrome

b.Young syndrome

c.Yellow –lymphedema syndrome

d.Williams-Campbell syndrome

e.Sinpson syndrome

6.All are true of permanent particulate emboli except

a. suspended in contrast medium

b. used in treatment of uterine leiomyomata

c. The level of occlusion depends on the size and type of particles chosen

d.safe in large arteriovenous communications

e. polyvinyl alcohol ia an example

7.All are true of embolisation except

a. Sclerosant materials are useful in varicoceles and low flow vascular malformations

b. gelatin sponge is used in traumatic injury to the internal iliac artery following pelvic trauma

c. Permanent particulate emboli are chosen for the treatment of benign or malignant tumours

d. Coils are best used in end arteries

e. Coils are not useful for packing the lumen of pseudoaneurysms

8.Liquid embolic agents is/are

a. absolute alcohol

b.polidocanol

c.hypertonic dextrose

d.isobutyl-2-cyanoacylate

e.all

9.Indication of embolisation is/are

a. a definitive treatment in nonmalignant lesions

b.may be used pre-operatively to reduce blood loss

c.may be used to alleviate symptoms

d. to manage visceral haemorrhage from the gastrointestinal tract or kidneys

e.all

10.Myocardial infarction imaging use

a. derivatives of tetracycline

b. derivatives of dicarboxylates

c. pyrophosphate.

d.^{99m}Tc-pyrophosphate and ^{111}In-labelled antimyosin

e.all

11.All are true regarding vascular rings except

a.surrounds the trachea and oesophagus causing compression

b.double aortic arch and right aortic arch with left ligamentum arteriosum are the most common complete vascular rings

c. Six pairs of arterial arches develop between paired ventral and dorsal aortas from approximately day 26

d. arterial arches are not all present at the same time

e. normally the right fourth arch develops into the aortic arch

12.All are true regarding double aortic arch except

a. both the right and left fourth arches persist

b. The right /posterior fourth arch is the larger in 75%

c. The normally positioned left/anterior fourth arch is anterior to the trachea.

d. The ligamentum arteriosum is positioned abnormally

e. The posterior/right fourth arch lies behind the oesophagus

13.---The mosty common of arch vessel anomalies is

a. Double aortic arch

b. Right aortic arch with aberrant left subclavian artery and left ligamentum arteriosum

c. Retro-oesophageal right subclavian artery with an otherwise normal left arch

d. Left aortic arch with right descending aorta and right ligamentum arteriosum

e. Right aortic arch with mirror-image branching and retro-oesophageal ligamentum arteriosum

14.All are true regarding bronchial vessels except

a.the bronchial arteries are distributed mainly in the central third of each lung

b. right bronchial artery usually shares its origin from the dorsolateral aorta with the first intercostal artery

c. the right bronchial artery courses in a long sharp 'hairpin' loop

d. The left bronchial artery originate from the descending aorta

e.Bronchial veins drain into the right atrium.

15.All are true regarding pulmonary physiology except

a. pulmonary arterial pressure rises equal to that in the right ventricle

during ventricular systole in the normal patients

b.mean pulmonary capillary pressure is 15 mmHg

c.mean pulmonary capillary wedge pressure is 5 mmHg

d. gas exchange is usually compromised by the presence of interstitial oedema alone

e. 'matched defects' noted in pneumonic consolidation on ventilation–perfusion imaging

16.All are true regarding pulmonary vessels except

a. . On plain radiograph and CT, the densities of the normal hilum are due mainly to lymphnode

b.The diameter of the artery is usually much the same as the diameter of the bronchus (4–5 mm).in anterior segment of upper lobe

c. Vessels in the first anterior interspace should not exceed 3 mm in diameter.

d. the lower lobe veins run more horizontally and the lower lobe arteries more vertically.

e.deep lymphatic channels run peribronchially and in the deep septa of the lungs.

17.All true regarding hila except

a. On plain radiograph and CT, the densities of the normal hilum are due mainly to blood vessels

b. Normal lymph nodes cannot be recognized as discrete structures,

c.the bronchial walls contribute little to the bulk of the hila,

d. there is relatively little signal generated from normal hilar structures on standard spin-echo sequences.

e. hilar points refers to point where the superior pulmonary vein crosses the descending lower lobe vein

18.All are true regarding soft tissue tumour of chest wall except

a.the most common primary benign tumour is neurofibroma

b.the most common primary malignant tumour is lipo/fibrosarcoma

c.Neurofibromas on CT characteristically have a lower density than muscle both before and after intravenous contrast medium

d.On MRI, neurofibromas give low to intermediate signal on T1-weighted images, high signal on T2w-weighted images and marked contrast enhancement

e. Lymphangiomas on CT have the features of a fluid-filled cyst with or without septation

19.The two main causes of rib notching

a. coarctation of the aorta and neurofibromatosis Type 2.

b. coarctation of the aorta and neurofibromatosis Type I.

c. osteoma and neurofibromatosis Type I.

d. coarctation of the aorta and muscular disorder.

e. coarctation of the aorta and marfan syndrome.

20.All are true regarding intrathoracic thyroidal mass except

a.continuous with thyroid gland in the neck

b. normal thyroid tissue within the mass shows a higher attenuation value than muscle before contrast

c. normal thyroid tissue within the mass shows a higher attenuation value than muscle after contrast

d. a benign and malignant mass on CT distinguishable in advanced stage

e. CT is less specific than nuclear medicine in diagnosing a thyroid origin

21. Mediastinal parathyroid tumours are probably best detected using

a.CT

b.MRI

c. ^{99m}Tc-sestamibi imaging

d.ultrasound

e.X- RAY

22.---All are true regarding *Strep. pneumoniae* pneumonia (pneumococcal pneumonia) except

a. a peripheral, homogeneous opacity with or without air bronchograms

b. commonly apical and solitary

c. Cavitation very unlikely

d. Parapneumonic effusion fairly common

e. total resolution within 2–6 weeks of treatment

23.Bulging fissures in chest x-ray is seen in

a. *Strep. pneumoniae pneumonia*

b. *Klebsiella pneumoniae pneumonia*

c. *Legionella pneumophila*

d. *Nocardia asteroids*

e. *Chlamydial pneumonia*

24.All are true regarding tracheobronchomegaly (Mounier–Kuhn disease) except
a. tracheal diameter of greater than 4 cm (measured 2 cm above the aortic arch) on CT scan
b. the immediate subglottic trachea has a normal diameter
c. associated with tracheal diverticulosis and bronchiectasis
d. corrugated outline of trachea on a plain radiograph
e. tracheal scalloping associated finding

25.Lunate shaped trachea is seen in
a. Tracheobronchomalacia
b. tracheobronchomegaly
c. Sabre-sheath trachea
d. Tracheobronchopathia osteochondroplastica
e. Wegener's granulomatosis

26.All are true regarding lung collapse except
a. upper lobe collapse often results in a shift of the superior mediastinum
b. lower lobe collapse often demonstrates elevation of the diaphragm
c. hilar elevation is sign of upper lobe collapse
d. ipsilateral main bronchus becomes more vertcally orientated than usual with significant upper lobe collapse
e. displacement of the anterior junctional line to the contralateral side of large collapse

27.All are indirect signs of lung collapse except
a. A convergent pattern of vascular reorientation near the hilum
b. shifting granuloma sign
c. the Luftsichel sign
d. juxtaphrenic peak of the diaphragm
e. Rib crowding

28.All are true regarding risk factors of bronchial carcinoma except
a.smoking increases risk of carcinoma 2-3 fold
b.exposure to asbestos, nickel and arsenic
c.interstitial pulmonary fibrosis
d.radiotherapy.
e.smoking most important factor

29.The incidence of which lung carcinoma is decreasing
a.adenocarcinoma
b.squamous cell carcinoma
c.bronchiolo-alveolar carcinoma
d.large cell carcinoma
e.small cell carcinoma

30.The imaging investigation most widely used to evaluate the primary lung tumour
a.chest x ray
b.CT
c.MRI
d.PET
e.CT-PET

31.All are true regarding interstitial lung disease except
a.HRCT provides insight into disease reversibility and prognosis.
b. A reticular pattern on CT almost always represents significant ILD

c. Smooth Interlobular septal thickening is seen in pulmonary oedema

d. irregular interlobular septal thickening is seen in alveolar proteinosis

e. Intralobular septal thickening seen in all ILDs

32.All are true regarding reticular pattern except

a.due to intelobular or intralobular thickening

b.subtle interlobulat thickening may cause ground glass opacity

c.honeycomb lung has cystic spaces surrounded by irregular walls

d. may produce bronchiectasis/bronchiolectasis

e. Intralobular septal thickening is most commonly noted in IPF

33.----All are true regarding rib fractures except

a.Fractures of the 1st to 3rd ribs is common in trivial trauma

b.fractures in posterior aspects of rib in children should raise the possibility of nonaccidental injury

c.More than 50% of acute fractures are missed on initial radiographs

d.Double fractures of three or more adjacent ribs are referred as 'flail chest'

e.In children, rib fractures are usually of the greenstick variety

34.An abnormally deep costophrenic sulcus sign is noted in

a.pneumothorax in supine position

b.pleural effusion in supine position

c.pleural effusion in decubitus position

d.pneumothorax in standing position

e.collapse of lower lobe

35.All are true regarding airspace diseases except

a. Wegener's granulomatosis may show cavitation on CT scan

b. In cryptogenic organizing pneumonia, areas of consolidation most pronounced in the periphery and lower zones of the lungs

c. in chronic eosinophilic pneumonia, the changes tend to be in the upper zones and parallel to the chest wall

d. transient and migratory opacities , unaccompanied by significant constitutional disturbance favour diagnosis of an eosinophilic pneumonia.

e. 'crazy-paving' pattern on CT is noted in alveolar proteinosis.

36.----All are true regarding pulmonary anatomy except

a. the respiratory bronchioles are the last purely conducting airways

b. the pores of Kohn link different alveolar units

c. the secondary pulmonary lobule is the smallest unit of lung bounded by connective tissue septa

d. the secondary pulmonary lobule is best seen sub-pleurally

e. The centrilobular arteries can be resolved HRCT in the normal lung

37.All are true regarding anatomy of right heart cavities except

a. the membranous septum lying above the tricuspid valve separates the left ventricle from the right atrium

b. the coronary sinus is the main draining vein of the heart

c. coronary sinus enter into the right atrium between the inferior vena cava and the pulmonary valve

d. the right coronary artery run in the anterior atrioventricular groove

e. infundibulum separates the right ventricular inflow and outflow

38.All are true regarding anatomy of left ventricles except

a. left ventricle is carrot shaped

b. The membranous septum lies between the right and noncoronary sinuses of Valsalva

c.The membranous septum provides the right attachment to the posterior leaflet of the mitral valve

d. The smooth muscular septum curves round the upper part of the left ventricle,

e. The smooth muscular septum forms part of the left border of the left ventricle

39.The fetal heart is most susceptible to rubella virus/thalidomide during

a.2-3 week of intrauterine life

b.3-5week of intrauterine life

c.5-7week of intrauterine life

d.7-9 week of intrauterine life

e.9-11week of intrauterine life

40.Which is not Endocardial cushions defect

a. Ostium primum defect /Tricuspid atresia

b. Endocardial atrioventricular defect

c. Ostium secundum defect

d. Cor triatrium

e. Ebstein's anomaly

41. Mitral annulus calcification appears on chest x ray as

a. C-shaped open ring/J-shaped

b. U-shaped open ring/J-shaped

c.Inverted U-shaped ring/J-shaped

d.X-shaped /J-shaped

e.Y-shaped/J-shaped

42. The cardinal radiological feature of rheumatic mitral valve disease is

a. righ atrial enlargement

b. left atrial enlargement

c. left ventricular enlargement

d. right ventricular enlargement

e.multi-chamber enlargement

43.ACC/AHA guidelines for coronary angiography are all except

a. Severe resting left ventricular dysfunction (LVEF < 35%)

b. High risk treadmill score (score ≥ 8)

c. Severe exercise left ventricular dysfunction (exercise LVEF < 35%)

d. Stress-induced large perfusion defect (particularly if anterior)

e. Stress-induced moderate size multiple perfusion defects

44.All are true regarding coronary artery angiography using MDCT except

a. allows reliable identification of patients who need invasive coronary angiography

b. may allow selection of those who need PCI at a specialist centre

c. A slow heart rate (<70 beats min) and freedom from artefact due to respiration or arrhythmia are essential

d. Beam hardening artefacts from calcification, stents or contrast medium in the superior vena cava can limit assessment of important segments of coronary arteries
e. navigator sequences, higher contrast imaging at 3T, and blood pool contrast agents have substantially improved image quality

45.All are true regarding lymphangiomyomatosis (LAM) and Langerhans cell histiocytosis (LCH) except
a.cyst usually round and relatively uniform in size and shape in LAM
b.unsual shapes of cysts in LCH
c.costophrenic angles usually spared in LAM
d.cysts larger and more numerous in lung apices in LCH
e.LAM almost exclusively in women

46.All are true regarding emphysema except
a.enlargement of air spaces distal to the respiratory bronchiole
b.inconspicous wall
c.centrilobular emphysema shows presence of multiple small lucencies,predominantly in upper lobes
d.panlobular emphysema results in an overall decrease in lung attenuation
e.bullous emphysema is often associated with centrilobular and paraseptal emphysema

47.All are true regarding pericardial disorder except
a. rapid accumulation of as little as 100–200 ml of fluid can cause a haemodynamically significant compression of the heart
b. attenuation values of a haemorrhagic effusion may overlap with the pericardial fluid found in patients with hypothyroidism
c. Malignant mesothelioma is the most common primary pericardial malignancy
d. A pericardial effusion is the most common finding in pericardial malignancy
e. Metastatic melanoma has low signal intensity on T1- and low on T2-weighted images

48.All are true regarding interpretation of cardiac scintigraphy except
a.Attenuation artefact may be due to female breast , breast augmentation, or a high diaphragm
b. Reverse distribution may be due to artefact
c. true reverse redistribution is the result of prolonged retention of tracer
d. true reverse redistribution may occur in an area of partial thickness infarction supplied by a patent artery after angioplasty or thrombolysis
e. Attenuation can be seen as reduced counts in the inferior wall, often in slim men

49.Resting coronary flow is normal until
a. the luminal area of a coronary artery is reduced by approximately 45–55% (equivalent to a 60–75% reduction in diameter)
b. resting coronary flow is normal until the luminal area of a coronary artery is reduced by approximately

85–90% (equivalent to a 60–75% reduction in diameter)

c. resting coronary flow is normal until the luminal area of a coronary artery is reduced by approximately 55–65% (equivalent to a 60–75% reduction in diameter)

d. resting coronary flow is normal until the luminal area of a coronary artery is reduced by approximately 65–75% (equivalent to a 60–75% reduction in diameter)

e. resting coronary flow is normal until the luminal area of a coronary artery is reduced by approximately 75–85% (equivalent to a 60–75% reduction in diameter)

50. All are true regarding stress techniques except

a. dipyridamole increases myocardial perfusion by between 100% and 200%

b. Adenosine increases mean coronary flow by 4.4 times the resting value

c. Dobutamine increases perfusion in normal myocardium approximately two-fold

d. Dobutamine may be used in patients with asthma

e. Adenosine has a very short plasma half-life

TEST PAPER 4(ANSWER)

1.-----d

In lung contusion radiographic opacities appear within 6 h of impact and typically clear within 3–10 d.Shadowing that increases in the days following admission is unlikely to be due to simple contusion and should be considered other possibilities, such as infection, aspiration, fat embolism, or acute respiratory distress syndrome .In pulmonary laceration there is haematoma, or pneumatocele, or both. **(CHAPTER 20 ,G)**

2.---d

The case showed the typical finding of lymphangitis carcinomatosis.**(CHAPTER 18 ,G)**

3.-----c

Between 6 and 16 weeks there is extensive branching of the respiratory tree. Between 16 and 28 weeks, multiple alveolar ducts arise from the respiratory bronchioles and the primitive alveoli form. True alveolar development extends from approximately 26 weeks gestation to term and continues for the first 2 years after birth, after which alveoli increase in size but not in number. **(CHAPTER 64,G)**

 4----689.----a **(CHAPTER 64 ,G)**

5.----e (Webb)

6----d

In large arteriovenous communications, permanent particulate emboli may pass through these into the venous system. (CHAPTER 28 G)

7----e

Coils are best used in end arteries where back filling is unlikely to occur .They are useful for packing the lumen of pseudoaneurysms or can be placed across the neck of a pseudoaneurysm to prevent 'front and back door' entry of blood. (CHAPTER 28,G)

8.-----e (CHAPTER 28 ,G)

9.-----e (CHAPTER 28,G)

10.-----e (CHAPTER 22,G)

11.----e

Normally the left fourth arch develops into the aortic arch. (CHAPTER 27 ,G)

12.-----d (CHAPTER 27 ,G)

13.---c

Retro-oesophageal right subclavian artery with an otherwise normal left arch is the most common of the arch vessel anomalies, occurring in about 0.5% of the population. (CHAPTER 27 ,G)

14.-----e

Bronchial veins drain into the left atrium.(CHAPTER 26 ,G)

15.-----d

Gas exchange is not usually compromised by the presence of interstitial oedema alone.(CHAPTER 26,G)

16.------a

On plain radiograph and CT, the densities of the normal hilum are due mainly to blood vessels (G)

17-----e

Hilar points refers to point where the superior pulmonary vein crosses the descending lower lobe artery.(G)

18.----a

The most common primary benign tumour of soft tissue of chest wall is lipoma.(G)

19.----b

The two main causes of rib notching are coarctation of the aorta and neurofibromatosis Type 1. (G)

20.----e

CT is almost as specific as nuclear medicine in diagnosing a thyroid origin Multiple masses are a feature of bengn multinodular goiter. (G)

21.----d

Mediastinal parathyroid tumours are probably best detected using ultrasound and if not readily apparent, by subsequent ^{99m}Tc-sestamibi imaging with CT or MRI only in selected cases (G)

22.----b

Strep. pneumoniae pneumonia (pneumococcal pneumonia) is commonly basal and solitary. Radiographic resolution is fairly rapid with some improvement commonly seen within 1 week and total resolution within 2–6 weeks. (Chapter 15,G)

23.-----b

Bulging fissures in chest x-ray is seen in *Klebsiella pneumoniae pneumonia* and signify significant exudative response. (Chapter 15,G)

24.----a

On CT a tracheal diameter of greater than 3 cm (measured 2 cm above the aortic arch) and diameters of 2.4 and 2.3 cm for the right and left bronchi, respectively, are diagnostic criteria of tracheobronchomegaly (Chapter 16,G)

25------a

Tracheobronchomalacia results from weakened tracheal cartilage rings . The increase in compliance is due to the loss of integrity of the wall's structural components and is particularly associated with damaged or destroyed cartilage. The coronal diameter of the trachea becomes significantly larger than the sagittal one, producing a lunate configuration. (Chapter 16,G)

26.----d

When upper lobe collapses significantly, the ipsilateral main bronchus becomes more horizontally orientated than usual, hence the bronchus intermedius and the left lower lobe bronchus swing laterally. When lower lobe collapses, each main bronchus is more vertically orientated than usual, with a medial swing of the bronchus intermedius on the right and the lower lobe bronchus on the left. .(Chapter 17, G)

27.----a

A divergent or parallel pattern of vascular reorientation seen near the hilum has been described in marked upper lobe collapse.Hyperexpansion may result in a change in position of lung lesions, such as granulomas resulting in the so-called shifting granuloma sign.The Luftsichel sign (from German, meaning air crescent) is due to the overinflated superior segment of the ipsilateral lower lobe occupying the space between the mediastinum and the medial aspect of the collapsed upper lobe, resulting in a paramediastinal translucency. Juxtaphrenic peak of the diaphragm, a useful ancillary sign of upper lobe collapse (or a combination of right upper and middle lobe collapse) refers to a small triangular density at the highest point of the dome of the hemidiaphragm, due to the anterior volume loss of the affected upper lobe resulting in traction and reorientation of an inferior accessory fissure. .(Chapter 17,G)

28.----a

Tobacco smoke is the most important causative agent imparting a 20–30-fold increased risk in smokers compared to non-smokers. (Chapter 18, G)

29.----b (Chapter 18, G)
30.----b (Chapter 18, G)
31.-----d

Interlobular septal thickening is usually described as smooth (seen in pulmonary oedema and alveolar proteinosis) or irregular

(lymphangitic spread of tumour). Intralobular septal thickening manifests as a fine reticular pattern on HRCT and is seen in all ILDs but most commonly in IPF. (Chapter 19, G)

32.----b

The intralobular septal thickening may be so fine that HRCT does not demonstrate discrete intralobular opacities but a generalized increase in lung density (ground-glass opacification). (Chapter 19, G)

33.----a

Fractures of the 1st to 3rd ribs imply severe trauma. (CHAPTER 20 ,G)

34.-----a

With supine radiographs, air collects anterior to the lung and there is no visible lung edge. In this situation a pneumothorax can produce an unusually sharp mediastinal border and hemidiaphragm and an abnormally deep costophrenic sulcus. . (CHAPTER 20,G)

35.-----b

In cryptogenic organizing pneumonia, areas of consolidation are most pronounced in the periphery and upper zones of the lungs.(CHAPTER 21,G)

36.----a

The terminal bronchioles are the last purely conducting airways of the bronchial tree and the region of lung subtended by a terminal bronchiole is termed the acinus (comprising the respiratory bronchioles, alveolar ducts, alveolar sacs and alveoli). The centrilobular arteries (with a diameter of 0.2 mm) can be resolved on high-resolution computed tomography (HRCT) in the normal lung, whereas normal bronchioles with a diameter below 2 mm are generally not seen. Infiltration of the interlobular interstitium by oedema fluid or malignant cells, or thickening by fibrosis, will render individual secondary pulmonary lobules visible on HRCT.(CHAPTER 21 ,G)

37.----c

Coronary sinus enter into the right atrium between the inferior vena cava and the tricuspid valve . (CHAPTER 22 ,G)

38.----c

The membranous septum provides the right attachment to the anterior leaflet of the mitral valve. (CHAPTER 22 ,G)

39.----b

The fetal heart develops between the second (total fetal length 2 mm) and eighth week of intrauterine life. It is during the third to fifth weeks of intrauterine life (when the forelimbs are developing) that the cardiac structures develop most actively and are therefore most susceptible to adverse external influence (e.g. rubella virus or drugs such as thalidomide). (CHAPTER 23 ,G)

40.---c

(CHAPTER 23,G)

41.----a

Mitral annulus calcification occurs in the angle between the left ventricle wall and the mitral valve cusps, and is readily recognized on the chest radiograph as a C-shaped open ring ; the gap in the ring occurs where the anterior mitral leaflet base is in contact with the posterior aortic valve ring. (CHAPTER 24,G)

42.----b

(CHAPTER 24.G)

43.----b

High risk treadmill score (score $\geq$11) is an indication of coronary angiography. (CHAPTER 25,G)

44.----a

With adequate image quality, MDCT allows reliable identification of patients who do not need coronary angiography. (CHAPTER 25,G)

45.----c

Costophrenic angles are usually spared in LCH (Webb)

46.----a

Emphysema is defined as a permanent abnormal enlargement of air spaces distal to the terminal bronchiole.(Webb)

47.----e

Metastatic melanoma may have high signal intensity on T1- and T2-weighted images.(Chapter 14,G)

48.----c

Reverse distribution is the term used to describe a defect in redistribution thallium images that is less apparent in the stress images. True reverse redistribution is the result of rapid washout of tracer. (CHAPTER 22,G)

49.----b

Resting coronary flow is normal until the luminal area of a coronary artery is reduced by approximately 85–90% (equivalent to a 60–75% reduction in diameter). (CHAPTER 22,G)

50.----a (CHAPTER 22,G)

TEST PAPER 5

1. All are true regarding hila except

a. The transverse diameter of the lower lobe arteries before their segmental divisions measure 9–16 mm on the normal postero-anterior (PA) chest radiograph

b. The posterior walls of the right main bronchus and the right upper lobe bronchus and bronchus intermedius as a thin stripe on lateral plain radiographs

c. The right pulmonary artery passes anterior to the major bronchi, whereas the left pulmonary artery arches superior to the left main bronchus

d. on the left, the left main bronchus lies between pulmonary artery and the superior pulmonary vein)

e. a rounded shadow of greater than 1 cm in angles (formed by the middle and right lower lobe bronchi on the right, and the upper and lower lobe bronchi on the left) on lateral x –ray is likely to be large end on vessel .

2. True regarding thymus

a. Before puberty' the thymus fills in most of the mediastinum in front of the great vessels

b. before puberty ,the gland varies greatly in size but is approximately symmetrical

c. In adults the thymus is bilobed or triangular in shape.

d. The maximum width and thickness of each lobe decreases with advancing age

e. Between the ages of 20 and 50, the maximum thickness of each lobe is up to 25 mm(CT)

3. All are true regarding rib lesions except

a. congenital rib anomalies are noted in Sprengel's deformity,but not noted in basal cell naevus syndrome

b. Destructive rib lesions occur most commonly in osteomyelitis or neoplastic disease

c. The most common malignant rib tumours are metastatic deposits and myeloma

d. the most common benign primary tumours of ribs is the cartilaginous tumours (chondromas, osteochondromas)

e. the least uncommon primary malignant tumours of rib is chondrosarcomas

4. All are true regarding sternum except

a. characteristic rib configuration (horizontal posteriorly and steeply oblique anteriorly) in pectus excavatum

b. neoplasms of the sternum are usually benign

c. the most common benign tumour is chondroma.

d. CT is the best investigation for imaging the sternum

e. pectus excavatum may be associated with Marfan's syndrome and atrial septal defect

5.The most common primary tumour of the anterior mediastinum in adults
a. lymphoma
b. thymoma
c.thymic carcinoid,
d. germ-cell tumour/teratoma
e.thymolipoma

6.All are true regarding thymoma except
a.The average age at diagnosis is approximately 50 years
b.late diagnosis in those who present with myasthenia gravis
c.up to 50% of patients with thymoma have myasthenia gravis,
 d. approximately 10–20% of patients with myasthenia gravis have a thymoma.
 e.may be associated with hypogammaglobulinaemia and red cell aplasia

7.All are true regarding pneumonia
a. *Legionella pneumophila* pneumonia has a tendency to give round and mass-like appearance
b.chest appearance of actinomycosis mimics bronchogenic carcinoma
c. Lymphadenopathy or chest wall involvement is seen in nocadia
d. The radiographic opacity in Chlamydial pneumonia characteristically clears very fast
e. Chlamydial pneumonia is one of the most common causes of community-acquired pneumonia.

8.All are true regarding actinomycosis of chest except
a.hilar lymphadenopathy
b. Cavitation and the appearance mimicking bronchogenic carcinoma
c. Pleural effusion, pleural thickening or empyema formation
d. extension of disease to the contiguous soft tissue or bones (as a periostitis)
e. homogeneous opacification as a lobar type pneumonia or mass

9.All are causes of bronchiectasis except
a. Sarcoidosis
b. Cystic fibrosis
c. Dyskinetic cilia syndrome
d. Allergic bronchopulmonary aspergillosis
e.Budd-chiari syndrome

10.All are causes of bronchiectasis except
a. yellow nail syndrome
b. Panbronchiolitis
c.Reigler s syndrome
d. α_1-Antitrypsin syndrome
e. Williams Campbell syndrome

11.All are signs of lung collapse except
a. shifting granuloma sign
b. Golden's S sign
c. the Luftsichel sign
d. juxtaphrenic peak of the diaphragm
e.Atoll sign

12.All are true regarding role of CT in lobar collapse except
a. identify an endobronchial or compressing lesion
b. collapsed lung usually enhances to a lesser degree than tumour with dynamic CECT
c. the S sign can be applied to collapse of all lobes on CT.

d. a localized convexity of adjacent fissure is highly suggestive of an underlying mass

e. the CT mucous bronchogram sign is highly suggestive of an obstructing lesion

13.All are true regarding peripheral bronchial carcinoma of lung except

a. Approximately 20% of bronchial carcinomas arise beyond the segmental bronchi

b. Lobulation

c. corona radiata

d. A peripheral line shadow or 'tail'

e. ill-defined edges notably in adenocarcinoma and bronchiole-alveolar carcinoma

14.All are true regarding bronchial carcinoma except

a. Pancoast's tumours may resemble apical pleural thickening

b. absolutely spherical, sharply defined, smooth-edged nodules due to carcinoma of the lung are rare

c. a peripheral line shadow or 'tail' may occur in both benign and malignant lesions

d. Adenocarcinoma is the most likely cell type to show cavitation

e. Calcification within bronchogenic carcinomas is identified on CT in 6–10% of cases

15.All conditions are characterized by profuse centrilobular nodules in HRCT except

a. Subacute hypersensitivity pneumonitis

b. Respiratory bronchiolitis–interstitial lung disease

c. Diffuse panbronchiolitis

d. Endobronchial spread of tuberculosis or bacterial pneumonia

e. sarcoidosis

16.All are true regarding ground-glass opacity on HRCT except

a. a generalized increase in opacity

b. obscure pulmonary vessels

c. due to partial filling of the airspaces and considerable thickening of the interstitium

d. bronchiectasis within ground glass usually indicate irreversibility of disease

e. subacute hypersensitivity pneumonitis is among the most common cause

17.All are true regarding injuries of the diaphragm except

a. Imaging plays great part in diagnosis of penetrating injuries

b. frontal impact to the abdomen cause tears at the musculotendinous junction in a posterolateral location

c. left-sided tears (72–88%) in blunt trauma more than right sided in clinical series

d. The chest radiograph is relatively insensitive in diagnosing diaphragmatic rupture

e. A nasogastric tube coiled within the left hemithorax is characteristic of a rupture

18.The key findings of diaphragm

rupture on CT are all except
a. discontinuity of the diaphragm
b. herniation of the abdominal organs into the chest
c. halo sign
d. dependent viscera sign
e. the 'collar sign'

19.All are true regarding ground glass opacity except
a.increase in lung density
b.presevation of bronchoalveolar markings on CT
c. obscuration of vessel markings on chest x ray
d. indicate disease within the airspaces only
e. 'black bronchus' sign

20.All causes increased permeability edema except
a. Drug-induced
b. cardiogenic edema
c. High altitude
d. Rapid re-expansion of collapsed lung
e. Intracranial disease

21.All are true regarding anatomy of left ventricles except
a. there is lack of a muscular infundibulum in the left ventricle
b.the upper left ventricle to reach up between the right coronary and left coronary sinuses of the aortic root
c. circumflex coronary artery (CX) run in the low attenuation fat of the anterior atrioventricular groove
d. the prominent crista terminalis (CT) in the wall of the right atrium is a normal structure commonly mistaken for a mass

e. The left anterior descending (LAD) coronary artery runs in the anterior interventricular groove

22.All are true regarding anatomy of heart except
a. The right ventricle forms the bulk of the front of the heart
b. The pulmonary valve lies cephalad, anterior and to the left of the aortic root
c. The posterior aspect of the heart is formed by the left atrium
d. The left ventricle lies posterior to the left atrium.
e. The left ventricle which forms the bulk of the left heart border

23.Which is not defect of bulbus cordis and ventricular outflow
a. Pulmonary stenosis (valve/infundibular)
b. Aortic stenosis (valve/subaortic)
c. Tetralogy of Fallot
d. Ventriculo-arterial discordance (uncorrected and corrected transposition)
e. Uhl's dysplastic right ventricle

24.Aortopulmonary window is defect of
a. Branchial (aortic) arches
b. Truncus arteriosus
c. Bulbus cordis
d. Endocardial cushions
e. Interventricular septum

25.All are features of left atrial enlargement except
a. straightening of the left heart border
b. 'double density' through the heart
c. large bulge immediately below the left main bronchus
d. displace the oesophagus backwards

e.upturning of apex

26.All are causes of tricuspid valve disease except

a. rheumatic disease

b. Ebstein's anomaly

c.alkaptonuria

d. endomyocardial fibrosis

e. Carcinoid syndrome

27.All are true regarding cardiac stress testing except

a. used to determine the functional consequences of CAD

b. Exercise, pacing, cold pressor testing are used as stress for testing

c. Perfusion defects are seen after the development of ischaemia

d. dobutamine/dipyridamole / adenosine are used as pharmacological agent for stress testing

e. the end-point of the test is usually the appearance of new wall motion abnormalities or a new perfusion defect.

28.All are true regading wall motion except

a. Wall motion scores are produced by dividing the ventricular wall into segments and assigning a value to each segment

b. Echocardiography is the most commonly used method

c. Tagging sequences and strain imaging technique has no significance for wall motion analysis

d. Scintigraphic and CMR techniques can be used for wall motion analysis

e. Wall motion may be reduced/absent/ paradoxical

29.Causes of pulmonary venous hypertension is/are

a. aortic coarctation

b. aortic stenosis

c.hypoplastic left heart

d.mitral valve disease

e.all

30.All are causes of pulmonary venous hypertention except

a.atrial myxoma

b.pulmonary veno-occlusive disease

c. Fibrosing mediastinitis

d. hypoplastic left heart

e.all

31.Which does not form complete vascular rings

a. Right aortic arch with aberrant left subclavian artery and left ligamentum arteriosum

b. Right aortic arch with mirror-image branching and retro-oesophageal ligamentum arteriosum

c. Left aortic arch with right descending aorta and right ligamentum arteriosum

d. Left aortic arch, right descending aorta and atretic right aortic arch

e. Retro-oesophageal right subclavian artery with an otherwise normal left arch

32.The most important study in patients with a suspected vascular ring

a.chest x ray

b. barium oesophagography

c. Computed tomography (CT)

d.magnetic resonance imaging (MRI)

e.digital subtraction angiography (DSA)

33.All are true regarding vascular anatomy of lower limb except

a. At the level of L4 the aorta divides into the common iliac arteries

b. At the level of the inguinal ligament, the external iliac artery becomes the common femoral artery

c. popliteal artery gives rise to the anterior and posterior tibial arteries and the peroneal artery

d. The anterior tibial artery is the most medial calf vessel whereas the posterior tibial artery is the most lateral vessel

e. the plantar arch is formed by the lateral plantar branch of the posterior tibial artery and the dorsalis pedis artery.

34. All are true regarding arterial disease affecting the lower extremity except

a. The most common cause of arterial occlusive disease in the lower extremity is atherosclerosis.

b. Patients with rest pain and tissue loss must be treated by angioplasty, stenting, or surgery.

c. arterial occlusive disease in diabetes involves mainly the distal vessels of the calf and feet

d. In the treatment of stenotic lesions of Iliac artery disease balloon angioplasty has a technical success rate approximating 100%

e. Stent is the mainstay of treatment for stenosis of the

superficial femoral artery

35.All are true of transient tachypnoea of the newborn except

a. prominent pulmonary interstitial markings,

b.fluid in the interlobar fissures and intrapleural space

c. pulmonary underaeration

d. usually symmetrical

e. radiographic resolution occurring by 48–72 h of

36.All are true regarding chest x ray of respiratory distress syndrome except

a. usually abnormal at 6 h

b. fine reticular and reticulogranular shodowing

c. increased aeration

d. bilaterally symmetrical disease

e. progressive loss of clarity of the diaphragmatic and cardiac contours

37.60 yrs old with hemoptysis was subjected to chest x ray and a solitary pulmonary nodule is noted in left mid lung field.Features on CT/PET favouring the diagnosis of malignancy are all except

a.irregular /speculated margin

b.laminated calcification

c.volume doubling time 30-400 days

d.enhancement more than 20HU

e.increased uptake of FDG

38. 25 year old man suffers from blunt trauma of chest after falling from motor-bike.His chest x-ray revealed fracture of 10 to 12 rib on right side.Next immediate appropriate management will be

a.wait and watch

b.pinning of the ribs

c.physiotherapy

d.stapping

e.usg of abdomen

39.Which emphysema is described as diffuse simplification of lung architecture ?

a. centrilobular emphysema

b. panlobular emphysema

c. bullous emphysema

d.paraseptal emphysema

e.cicatricial emphysema

40.Factors which favour paraseptal emphysema over honeycombing are all except

a.typically marginated by thin linear opacities extending to the pleural surface

b.usually occur in single layer at the pleural surface

c.predominate in upper lobe

d.disruption of lobular architecture

e.unassociated with significant fibrosis

41.All may be causes V/Q scan leading to false diagnosis of pulmonary embolism

a. pulmonary artery wall causes, e.g. vasculitis, infection, irradiation

b. vascular malformations, e.g. arterial agenesis, arteriovenous malformations, surgical shunts

c. extrinsic compression of vasculature, e.g. from hilar adenopathy or tumour

d. pulmonary artery luminal block, e.g. from non-thrombotic material or tumour

e.all

42.All are true regarding endoleaks except

a. Type I is is due to failure to obtain a seal either proximally or distally

b. type 1 is left as such and resolve itself

c. Type II is caused by retrograde flow into the sac from lumbar or inferior mesenteric arteries

d. Type III is due to a failure of the stent graft material

e. Type IV is due to graft porosity

43.All are true except

a. aortic sinus aneurysms may be congenital, particularly in Asian populations

b. aortic sinus aneurysms may be seen in Marfan's syndrome

c. The most common site of aortic sinus aneurysms is from the right aortic sinus into the right ventricle or right atrium

d. More patients with Inflammatory aneurysms (IAAAs) have a positive family history of aneurysms than noninflammatory aneurysms

e. Steroid therapy is of no use in treatment of inflammatory aneurysm

44.A scoring system for assessment pulmonary effect of cystic fibrosis based on thin section CT is named as

a. Crispin–Norman

b. Shwachmann

c. Bhalla

d.snowden

e.sinha

45.All are true except
a.random distribution of nodules is seen in miliary tuberculosis
b.Tree-in –bud almost always indicates the presence of bronchiolar infection
c.centrilobular nodules are usually centered 5-10 mm from pleural surface
d.random nodules are distributed in a diffuse and uniform manner
e.perilymphatic distribution noted in military tuberculosis

46.All are true regarding ground glass opacity except
a.hazy increase in lung opacity
b.results from volume averaging of morphological abnormalities on HRCT
c.no obscuration of vessels
d.dark appearance of air-filled bronchi
e.insignificant HRCT finding

47.HRCT finding in active tuberculosis
a.patchy unilateral or bilateral airspace consolidation
b.cavitation—thin or thick-walled
c.scattered airspace (acinar) nodules
d.centrilobular branching structures/tree-in bud appearance
e.all

48.Factors that favour military nodules over nodules seen in endobronchial spread is/are
a.smaller size (1-3mm)
b.uniform diameter
c.even distribution
d.lack of bronchial wall thickening
e.all

49.All are features of pericardial effusion except
a. The epicardial fat pad 'sign'
b. Filling in of the retrosternal space
c.effacement of the normal cardiac borders
d.development of a 'flask'/'water bottle' cardiac configuration,
e.unilateral hilar overlay

50.All are true regarding chronic pericarditis except
a. a pericardial calcification and restriction of diastolic filling
b. The left ventricle tends to be of reduced volume and has a narrow tubular configuration
c. the most common cause is probably tuberculosis or fungal aetiology (outside USA)
d. Pericardial thickening(>4mm) is seen in up to 88% of confirmed cases
e. involves the entire pericardium in most of cases

TEST PAPER 5(ANSWER)

1.---- e
On lateral chest radiographs the angles between the middle and right lower lobe bronchi on the right, and the upper and lower lobe bronchi on the left, do not contain any large end-on vessels; a rounded shadow of greater than 1 cm in these angles is therefore unlikely to be a normal vessel.

The pulmonary veins are similar on the two sides. The superior pulmonary vein is the anterior structure in the upper and mid hilum on both sides.

On the right the superior pulmonary vein is separated from the central bronchi by the lower division of the right pulmonary artery, whereas on the left the superior pulmonary vein is separated from the pulmonary artery by the bronchial tree. (G)

2.----e
Between the ages of 20 and 50, the average thickness as measured by CT decreases from 8–9 mm to 5–6 mm, the maximum thickness of each lobe being up to 15 mm. These diameters are greater on MRI, presumably because MRI demonstrates the thymic tissue even when it is partially replaced by fat. On MRI, sagittal images demonstrate the gland to be 5–7 cm long in its craniocaudal dimension. (G)

3.----a
Congenital rib anomalies are noted in basal cell naevus syndrome and Sprengel's deformity. **(G)**

4.----a
Neoplasms of the sternum are usually malignant (myeloma, chondrosarcoma, lymphoma or metastatic carcinoma). (G)

5.---b
The most common primary tumour of the anterior mediastinum in adults. **(G)**

6.----b
The average age at diagnosis is approximately 50 years, earlier in those who present with myasthenia gravis. Thymomas are rare under 20 years of age and extremely unusual below the age of 15. **(G)**

7.---d
The radiographic opacity characteristically clears slowly and persistent changes at 3 months are not uncommon in Chlamydial pneumonia. (Chapter 15,G)

8.----a
Pleural effusion, pleural thickening or empyema formation, and extension of disease to the contiguous soft tissue or bones (as a periostitis) set actinomyocotic pneumonia apart from the usual bacterial types. (Tuberculosis and nocardiosis may have a similar appearance.) At CT, scattered peripheral areas of homogeneous consolidation with central low attenuation and adjacent pleural

thickening are suggestive of actinomycosis. (Chapter 15,G)

9.----e (Chapter 16,G)

10.-----c (Chapter 16,G)

11.---e

The Golden's S sign refers to the S shape (or more accurately, reverse S on the right) of the fissure due to the combination of collapse and mass centrally resulting in a focal convexity with a concave outline peripherally. Although the sign was originally described in the right upper lobe, it can be seen in any lobe. (Chapter 17,G)

12.-----b

Collapsed lung usually enhances to a greater degree than tumour with dynamically contrast-enhanced CT. (Chapter 17, G)

13.-----a

Approximately 40% of bronchial carcinomas arise beyond the segmental bronchi, and in 30% a peripheral mass is the sole radiographic finding.(Chapter 18,G)

14.-----d

Squamous cell carcinoma is the most likely cell type to show cavitation.(Chapter 18, G)

15.----e

Nodules within the lung interstitium, especially those related to the lymphatic vessels, are seen in the interlobular septa, subpleural and peribronchovascular regions; a distribution seen most commonly in sarcoidosis but also in lymphangitis carcinomatosa. A random distribution of very small well-defined nodules is seen in patients with haematogenous spread of tuberculosis, pulmonary metastases, pneumoconiosis and rarely in pulmonary sarcoidosis .(Chapter 19, G)

16.----b

The definite identification of dilated airways within areas of ground glass is usually an indication of fine fibrosis and thus usually indicates irreversible disease. But in organizing pneumonia,dilated airways that are present within areas of ground glass in the acute setting, may completely resolve following successful treatment. (Chapter 19,G)

17.-----a

Penetrating injuries of diaphragm are normally diagnosed by surgical exploration in the region of the wound, including laparoscopic or thoracoscopic techniques. Imaging plays little part in their diagnosis. . (CHAPTER 20 ,G)

18.----c

The 'collar sign' refrs to Constriction of the stomach or colon as it passes through the tear of diaphragm . Dependent viscera sign refers to an abnormally posterior location of organs like spleen /liver due to the lack of the normal support from the diaphragm (CHAPTER 20 ,G)

19.-----d
Ground glass opacity indicate disease within the airspaces and/or the interstitium.It may or may not be an associated with air bronchogram. In cases of uncertainty, comparison of the (air) density within airways with that of lung parenchyma (the 'black bronchus' sign) may be useful, normally the two densities are roughly comparable. .(CHAPTER 21 ,G)

20.-----b
Cardiogenic edema causes hydrostatic edema. .(CHAPTER 21,G)

21-----c
Circumflex coronary artery (CX) run in the low attenuation fat of the posterior atrioventricular groove. (CHAPTER 22,G)

22.-----d
The left ventricle lies anterior to the left atrium. . (CHAPTER 22 ,G)
23.-----e
Uhl's dysplastic right ventricle is defect of Interventricular septum and ventricles. (CHAPTER 23,G)

24.----b
(CHAPTER 23 ,G)

25.-----e
(CHAPTER 24 ,G)

26.-----c
(CHAPTER 24,G)

27.-----c
The use of stress testing is dependent on a cascade of events when there is a flow limiting stenosis. Perfusion defects are seen before the development of ischaemia, causes a reduction in

wall motion and myocardial thickening. These events precede ECG changes and are therefore more sensitive for detecting ischaemia than the conventional ECG-based exercise test. (CHAPTER 25,G)

28.-----c
Tagging sequences and strain imaging techniques can increase the accuracy and reproducibility of wall motion analysis. (CHAPTER 25,G)

29.----e
(CHAPTER 26,G)

30.----e
(CHAPTER 26,G)

31.----e
(CHAPTER 27 ,G)

32.-----b
Barium oesophagography is the most important study in patients with a suspected vascular ring, and it is diagnostic in the vast majority of cases. (CHAPTER 27 ,G)

33.----d
The anterior tibial artery is the most lateral calf vessel whereas the posterior tibial artery is the most medial. (CHAPTER 28,G)

34.----e
Angioplasty is the mainstay of treatment for stenosis of the superficial femoral artery. . (CHAPTER 28 ,G)

35.----c
In severe cases of TTN , the radiographic appearance is that of alveolar oedema or a reticular granular appearance similar to that of respiratory distress

syndrome of the newborn, with the only difference being that pulmonary aeration is normal to slightly increased. **(CHAPTER 64 ,G)**

36.----c

There is normal to decreased aeration of the lungs as compared to TTN, where there is increased aeration. **(CHAPTER 64,G)**

37.---b

Calcification occurs in upto 14% of lung cancer.The calcification is amorphous while diffuse solid ,central punctuate,laminated or popcorn-like calcification are noted in benign lesions. Lung cancers typically double in volume (an increase of diameter of 26% in diameter) between 30-400days (average 240 days).An absence of growth over a 2-year period is usually a reliable feature of benign nodule. Cavitation in malignant nodule shows thick irregular wall (thin and smooth wall in benign nodule) (Hagga)

38.-----e

Fractures of the 10th to 12th ribs, are associated with injuries to the liver, spleen, or kidneys. Further imaging of these organs is mandatory when such fractures are detected.(G)

39.-----b (Webb)

40.-----d

Honeycombing is associated with disruption of lobular architecture .(Webb)

41.-----e

(CHAPTER 6,G)

42.-----b

Type I is the most dangerous and is due to failure to obtain a seal either proximally or distally. This should not be left and is usually solved with a moulding balloon and/or a cuff. The term endotension (Type V) is applied where there is sac expansion in the absence of a recognizable Type I to IV endoleak. .(CHAPTER 27,G)

43.----e

Steroid therapy has been used to control the inflammatory process.(CHAPTER 27 ,G)

44.-----c

(CHAPTER 64 ,G)

45.-----e (Webb)

46.-----e

Ground glass opacity is a highly significant finding,as it often indicates the presence of an ongoing ,active and potentially treatable process.(Webb)

47.----e (Webb)

48.-----e(Webb)

49.-----e

bilateral hilar overlay is a feature of pericardial effusion .On chest radiograph sudden increase in the size of the cardiac silhouette without specific chamber enlargement suggests the diagnosis of pericardial effusion. The epicardial fat pad 'sign' is positive when, visualized in the lateral projection, an anterior pericardial stripe (bordered by epicardial fat posteriorly and mediastinal fat anteriorly) is thicker than 2 mm. This sign is diagnostic of pericardial thickening or fluid. (Chapter 14,G)

50.----b
Both CT and MRI may show the secondary effects of constriction on the central cardiovascular structures. The right ventricle tends to be of reduced volume and has a narrow tubular configuration. A sigmoid-shaped interventricular septum or prominent leftward convexity of the septum may be seen. The right atrium, superior and in particular inferior venae cavae, and hepatic veins may be dilated. Hepatomegaly and ascites may be seen. (Chapter 14,G)

TEST PAPER 6

1.40 yrs male patient,engaged in heavy metal mining for last 15yrs, started complaining of cough and shortness of breath .X ray shows multiple small nodules in both lung field ,most numerous in upper lobes and perihilar regions .HRCT shows diffuse bilateral nodules that are centrilobular /subpleural in location .There is no nodules in relation to thickened interlobular septa.The most likely diagnosis is
a.CWP
b.silicosis
c.sarcoidosis
d.PLC
e.asbestosis

2.A young female patient had early morning stiffness and symmetrical arthritis of small joints.The patient is RA +.This patient is associated with respiratory problem .Which is uncommon finding on HRCT of such patients is
a.lower lung zone and posterior predominance
b.bronchiectasis
c.fibrosis
d. ground glass opacity
e.small centrilobular nodules (follicular bronchiolitis)

3.All are true regarding respiratory distress syndrome except
a. 50% of neonates born between 26 and 28 weeks develop
b. Very small infants(less than 25 weeks gestation)develop typical RDS
c. RDS is due to a deficiency of alveolar surfactant
d. antenatal corticosteroid administration useful
e. hyaline membrane disease stains pink with standard histological preparations

4.All are true regarding treatment of respiratory distress syndrome except
a. Surfactant acts synergistically with antenatal corticosteroid therapy to reduce the severity of RDS
b. Pressures in the range of 2–6 cmH$_2$O are used during CPAP and peak pressures between 12 and 26 cmH$_2$O are commonly used during IPPV.
c. The efficiency of high-frequency oscillatory ventilation is normally measured by radiological assessment of the degree of lung filling
d. The right diaphragm should be seen to lie at a level between the posterior ends of the eighth and

ninth ribs
e. complications of barotrauma resolve more quickly with High-frequency ventilation than with conventional ventilation

5.All are true except
a. The coeliac arteries and the superior mesenteric artery (SMA) usually arise at the level of T12 and L1, respectively
b. inferior mesenteric artery (IMA) arises at the level of L3
c. Upper gastro-intestinal (GI) haemorrhage is defined as bleeding proximal to the duodenal–jejunal flexure
d. the superior and inferior mesenteric arteries donot anastomose
e. The coeliac artery and SMA anastomose with each other via the pancreaticoduodenal arcades

6.All are true of GI angiography except
a. angiography for mesenteric haemorrhage is performed if endoscopy is negative
b. angiography can detect active bleeding at a rate of 0.5 ml /min
c. particulate emboli are used in the upper GI tract where there is good collateral supply
d. Red cell scintigraphy is less sensitive than angiography
e. The only direct sign of haemorrhage is contrast extravasation into the bowel lumen

7.All are true regarding barium imaging of double aortic arch except
a. persistent posterior compressions of the trachea
b. persistent posterior compressions of the oesophagus
c. The right indentation in esophagus is usually slightly higher than the left
d. the posterior indentation in esophagus is usually wide
e. The right indentation in esophagus courses in a downward direction from right to left

8.All are true regarding aortic coarctation except
a. the aortic isthmus (95% of cases) most common site
b. Eighty per cent of patients are male.
c. In females, coarctation is associated with Turner's syndrome
d. The infantile type of coarctation is usually proximal to the ductus arteriosus
e. collaterals develop in utero in infantile variety

9.Which sign is often the first recognized radiological sign of pulmonary venous hypertension
a. upper lobe venous diversion
b. interstitial (Kerley B) lines
c. perihilar haze
d. peribronchial cuffing
e. interstitial (Kerley A) lines

10.All are true regarding Kerley B lines except
a. 1 cm or less in length
b. found predominantly in the mid zones

c.peripheral location and parallel to each other but

d.at right angles to the pleural surface

e. as a result of fluid accumulation in interlobular septa

11.The Macklin effect is related to

a.pneumomediastinum

b.pneumothorax

c.pneumopericardium

d.pericardial effusion

e.pneumoperitoneum

12.All are true regarding Kerley B lines except

a. due to fluid in the interlobular septa

b. typically 1–2-mm wide

c.typically 30–60-mm long

d. mainly seen in the sub-pleural lung,

e.parallel to the pleural surface

13.All are true regarding Kerley A lines except

a. up to 80–100 mm long

b.occasionally angulated

c.cross the inner 0ne -thirds of the lung

d.varying directions

e. point medially towards the hilum

14. All are true regarding anatomy of heart except

a.left anterior oblique plane forms the septal plane of the heart

b. The aortic valve lies in the centre of the cardiac mass

c. the left main (LMCA) and right (RCA) coronary arteries arise from the aortic root about 1 cm caudal to the valve ring

d. ramus intermedius artery ia a diagonal branch arises from the bifurcation of the LMCA

e. The posterior descending coronary artery lies in the postero-inferior interventricular groove

15. All are true regarding anatomy of heart except

a.the right coronary artery passes anteriorly in the right (anterior) atrioventricular groove

b. the circumflex branch of the left coronary artery lies in the left (posterior) atrioventricular groove

c. the atrioventricular and posterior interventricular grooves intersect on the postero-inferior surface of the heart at the crus of the heart

d. The coronary artery that reaches the crux and supplies the posterior interventricular branch is termed the dominant coronary artery

e. the dominant coronary artery is usually the left coronary artery (85%).

16.All are true regarding cardiac anatomy except

a. formation of dextro loop and almost always clockwise rotation during devepolment

b.fetal IVC carries partially oxygenated from the fetal placenta

c.fetal systemic arteries receives blood via the PDA only

d. Oxygenated blood is carried by the umbilical vein (UV) through the ductus venosus (DV) into the right atrium

e. within a few days of postnatal life, the right-to-left shunting is abolished through both the foramen ovale and PDA.

17. All are congenital cyanotic heart disease except
a. tetralogy of Fallot
b. uncorrected transposition of great arteries (UTGA).
c. common atria and common ventricles
d. PDA
e. persistent truncus arteriosus

18. All are true regarding cardiac enlargement except
a. increasing curvature of the right heart border suggest of right atrial enlargement
b. enlargement of right atrial appendage seen as increased retrosternal density in the lateral projection
c. Rounding of the cardiac apex may suggest right ventricular hypertrophy
d. Localized prominence of the ascending aorta may indicate post-stenotic dilatation
e. In aneurysmal enlargement, the left atrium reaches to within an inch or so of the chest wall

19. Probably the most accurate method for determining ventricular mass is
a. Echo
b. CMR
c. MDCT
d. PET
e. Chest x ray

20. All are most common causes of ground glass opacity except
a. cystic bronchiectasis
b. acute respiratory distress syndrome (ARDS)

c. acute interstitial pneumonia (AIP)
d. non-specific interstitial pneumonia (NSIP)
e. *Pneumocystis jirovecii (carinii)* pneumonia in AIDS patients

21. All are true regarding ILD except
a. mosaic attenuation pattern refers to regional attenuation differences demonstrated on HRCT
b. small airways disease, occlusive vascular disease and infiltrative lung disease all cause mosaic attenuation
c. A nodular pattern is a feature interstitial disease only
d. A reticular pattern on CT almost always represents significant ILD
e. Intralobular septal thickening is noted most commonly in IPF

22. All are true regarding bronchogenic tumour except
a. cavity with irregular wall and usually =/>8mm thick
b. Air bronchograms and pseudocavitation may be particularly seen in squamous cell carcinoma
c. may be associated with bronchocele
d. nodule with Ground-glass attenuation is associated with a greater risk of malignancy
e. bronchiolo-alveolar carcinoma may present as a purely ground-glass opacity.

23. Features suggesting that pneumonia may be secondary to an obstructing neoplasm are all

except
a. the Golden S sign
b. unchanged persistence for longer than 2–3 weeks and recurrence in the same lobe
c. irregular stenosis in a mainstem or lobar bronchus
d. rarely associated with hilar adenopathy
e. Mucus-filled dilated bronchi visible within collapsed lobes

24.The CT mucous bronchogram sign is noted in all except
a. allergic bronchopulmonary aspergillosis
b.asthma
c.cystic fibrosis
d. an obstructing lesion causing lobar collapse
e.alveolar proteinosis

25.Drowned lobe refers to
a.collapsed lobe due to central obstructing lesion
b.consolidated lobe
c. collapsed lobe due to pleural effusion
d.collapsed lobe due to cicatrisation
e.collapsed lobe due to external compression

26.All are x ray features of bronchiectasis except
a. single thin lines or as parallel line opacities (tramlines)
b. poorly defined ring or curvilinear opacities
c. tubular or ovoid opacities of variable size

d. Pulmonary vessels may appear increased in size and may be distinct
e. multiple thin-walled ring shadows often containing air–fluid levels

27.The fallen lung sign is noted in
a. complete rupture of a mainstem bronchus
b.hydatid cyst of lung
c.diaphragmatic rupture
d.Cirrhosis of liver
e.asplenia

28.All are features of bronchial dilatation on CT except
a. lack of tapering of bronchial lumina
b. internal bronchial diameter less than that of the adjacent pulmonary artery
c. visualization of bronchi within 1 cm of the costal pleura or abutting the mediastinal pleura
d. visualization of bronchi abutting the mediastinal pleura
e. mucus-filled dilated bronchi

29.All are true of thymoma except
a. Most thymomas (90%) arise in the upper anterior mediastinum
b. may contain cysts and Calcification
c. usually gives rise to an asymmetrical focal swelling.
d. Thymomas usually show homogeneous density and no enhancement
e. transpleural spread in invasive thymoma

30.All are true regarding thymic mass except
a. thymic carcinoid may produce Cushing's syndrome
b. thymic hyperplasia is associated with myasthenia gravis and thyrotoxicosis
c. Stress,steroid or antineoplastic drug therapy may cause thymus atrophy
d. CT features of thymic carcinoid is entirely different from those of thymoma
e. Thymolipomas mould themselves to the adjacent mediastinum and diaphragm

31.All are true regarding pleural effusion except
a. Bilateral pleural effusions tend to be transudates
b. Right-sided effusions are typically associated with ascites, heart failure and liver abscess
c. left-sided effusions are typically associated with pancreatitis, pericarditis, oesophageal rupture and aortic dissection.
d.Massive effusions are most commonly due to malignant disease, particularly metastases (lung or breast),
e. transudative bilateral effusions are seen with metastatic disease, lymphoma

32. All are true regarding x- ray features of pleural effusions except
a. it initially tends to collect in the posterior costophrenic angles
b.lateral costophrenic angles become blunted on 200–500 ml of pleural effusion

c. curvilinear upper margin higher laterally than medially in PA view
d. mesothelioma may cause massive effusion with no mediastinal shift
e. diaphragmatic inversion in massive effusion

33.A bullae is defined as a sharply demarcated area of emphysema measuring
a. 1 cm or more
b.2 cm or more
c.0.5 cm or more
d.1.5 cm or more
e.2.5 cm or more

34.Strings of Pearls is noted in
a.cylindrical bronchietasis
b.varicose bronchietasis
c.cystic bronchiectasis
d.traction bronchiectasis
e.honeycombing

35.Two most common complete vascular rings are
a. double aortic arch and right aortic arch with left ligamentum arteriosum
b. double aortic arch Right aortic arch with retro-oesophageal ligamentum arteriosum
c. right aortic arch with left ligamentum arteriosum and Right aortic arch with retro-oesophageal ligamentum arteriosum
d. Left aortic arch with right ligamentum arteriosum and double aortic arch
e. double aortic arch and Right aortic arch with retro-oesophageal ligamentum arteriosum

36.Erasmus syndrome refers to
a. the association of silicosis and

rheumatoid arthritis
b. the association of silicosis and systemic sclerosis
c. the association of CWP and rheumatoid arthritis
d. the association of Berrylosis and rheumatoid arthritis
e. the association of CWP and systemic sclerosis

37.The most common manifestation of asbestos exposure is
a. Benign pleural effusions
b. Pleural plaques
c. Diffuse pleural thickening
d. Round atelectasis
e. Asbestosis

38.Which shows high incidence with Down's syndrome
a.AVSD
b.ASD
c.VSD
d.PDA
e.TOF

39.The most common congenital heart lesions
a.VSD
b.ASD
c.PDA
d.TAPVC
e.TOF

40.Radiopharmaceuticals used in myocardial perfusion study is/are
a. thallous chloride
b. ^{99m}Tc-2-methoxy-isobutyl-isonitrile (MIBI),
c. ^{99m}Tc-1, 2-bis[bis(2-ethoxyethyl) phosphino] ethane (tetrofosmin)
d. ^{99m}Tc-teboroxime
e.all

41.All are true regarding radiopharmaceuticals except
a. MIBI and tetrofosmin are essentially fixed in the myocardium with no redistribution
b. Imaging starts within 30–60 min of injection of thallium and should be completed within 30 min
c. Thallium washes out of the myocardium at a slower rate in underperfused than normally perfused myocardium
d. Regional defects noted in reduced perfusion in viable myocardium and/or a reduced amount of viable myocardium,
e. Areas of infarction show defects on both stress and rest images

42.All are true regarding imaging of pericardial disease except
a. Ultrasound is the most commonly used investigation in the initial evaluation of pericardial disease
b. Computed tomography is the best investigation for localizing, characterizing and demonstrating the extent of a collection or mass in the acute setting
c. Computed tomography is highly sensitive for the detection of pericardial calcification
d. Magnetic resonance imaging can assess pericardial disease but not its impact on cardiac function
e. Differentiating pericardial fluid from thickening may occasionally be difficult on CT.

43.All are true regarding developmental anomalies of pericardial disease except

a. the most common form of congenital absence of pericardium is complete absence of the left pericardium

b. Complete absence of the pericardium is usually asymptomatic

c. displacement of the heart into the right chest is x-ray feature of complete absence of the left pericardium

d. most Pericardial cysts occur in the right cardiophrenic angle

e. intrapericardial bronchogenic cysts are rare

44.All are true regarding complications of myocardial infarction except

a. cardiac rupture is an uncommon complication

b. true aneurysm shows enhancement on DE-MRI

c. Postinfarction VSD is most frequently seen towards the apex

d. Acute mitral regurgitation may be caused by papillary muscle dysfunction

e. TOE is probably the most reliable technique for diagnosing ventricular thrombus

45.All are role of IVUS except

a. widely used to assess the results of PCI

b. for assessing the adequacy of stent deployment

c. enables direct measurements of lumen dimensions

d. allows characterization of atheroma size, calcification ,

plaque ulceration and lesion composition

e. Adequacy of arterial flow cannot be assessed with intravascular Doppler.

46.Which of following indicate high probability of pulmonary embolism according to PIOPED STUDY

a. ≤ 3 small perfusion defects with a normal chest radiograph

b. > 3 small perfusion defects with a normal chest radiograph

c. Solitary moderate perfusion defect (matched/mismatched) with a normal chest radiograph

d. ≥ 2 large ventilation–perfusion mismatches with a normal chest radiograph

e. Solitary perfusion defect considerably smaller than the chest radiograph defect

47.Carney complex is associated with

a. cardiac myxoma

b. rhabdomyomas

c.fibromas

d.lipoma

e.fibroelastosis

48.Imaging features of cardiac myxoma are all except

a. left atrial enlargement

b.low signal intensity on GRE

c. higher signal intensity on T2-weighted sequences

d. A no contrast enhancement

e. may show the mobility on cine MRI

49.The most common paediatric primary cardiac tumour

a. Rhabdomyomas

b.myxoma

c.fibroma

d.lipoma

e.sarcomas

50.Whorls of calcium is characteristic of which cardiac tumour

a. Rhabdomyomas

b.myxoma

c.fibroma

d.lipoma

e.sarcomas

TEST PAPER 6(ANSWER)

1.----b
Any occupation that disturbs the earth's crust or exposes the worker to the use or processing of silica-containing rock or sand has potential risks of silicosis. Mining, tunnelling through rock, quarrying, stone cutting and foundry work, are potentially hazardous occupations. Coal worker's pneumoconiosis (CWP) is a consequence of the inhalation of coal dust.Egg-shell calcification of hilar lymph node is almost pathognomonic of silicosis and is found in 5% cases Beaded septa is seen in PLC and sarcoidosis.(webb)

2.----e (Webb)

3.-----b
Very small infants, less than 25 weeks gestation, often do not develop typical RDS. Approximately 50% of neonates born between 26 and 28 weeks and 20–30% of neonates born at 30–31 weeks of gestation develop RDS. **(CHAPTER 64 ,G)**

4.-----e
High-frequency ventilation allows adequate gas exchange at lower peak inspiratory pressures and complications of barotrauma resolve more quickly than with conventional ventilation. **(CHAPTER 64 ,G)**

5.----d
The superior and inferior mesenteric arteries anastomose via the middle colic branch of the SMA and left colic branch of the IMA, just proximal to the splenic flexure. (CHAPTER 28,G

6.----d
Red cell scintigraphy is more sensitive than angiography and can detect bleeding rates as low as 0.1 ml min⁻, but is not able to localize precisely the site of haemorrhage. (CHAPTER 28,G)

7.-----a
A double aortic arch produces bilateral and posterior compressions of the oesophagus, which remain constant regardless of peristalsis. The right indentation is usually slightly higher than the left and the posterior one is usually rather wide and courses in a downward direction from right to left. Where the right subclavian artery takes a retro-oesophageal course there is a posterior defect slanting upward from left to right. The posterior defect in these cases is usually not as broad as that found in a double aortic arch. (CHAPTER 27 ,G)

8.-----e

The infantile type of coarctation is usually proximal to the ductus arteriosus and 50% are associated with other congenital heart defects such as bicuspid aortic valve, ventricular septal defect (VSD), or hypoplastic left heart syndrome. Cystic medial necrosis of the aorta is also associated. At birth the ductus arteriosus closes, resulting in reduced blood supply to the distal aorta, which is perfused up to this time via the duct. The consequent increased strain on the heart leads to heart failure, as no collateral pathways are required in utero.(CHAPTER 27,G)

9.-----a (CHAPTER 26 ,G)

10.-----b

Kerley B lines are shorter (1 cm or less) interlobular septal lines, found predominantly in the lower zones peripherally, and parallel to each other but at right angles to the pleural surface. (CHAPTER 26 ,G)

11.-----a

In more than 95% of cases, pneumomediastinum results from alveolar rupture due to lung trauma or positive-pressure ventilation or both. Following alveolar rupture, air tracks through the pulmonary interstitium along peribronchovascular sheaths and into the mediastinum, a process known as the Macklin effect.). (CHAPTER 20 ,G)

12.----e

Kerley B lines are perpendicular to the pleural surface. (CHAPTER 21,G)

13.-----c

In comparison to Kerley B lines, Kerley A lines are longer (up to 80–100 mm), occasionally angulated and cross the inner two-thirds of the lung in varying directions but tend to point medially towards the hilum. (CHAPTER 21,G)

14.----c

The left main (LMCA) and right (RCA) coronary arteries arise from the aortic root about 1 cm cephalad to the valve ring. (CHAPTER 22,G)

15.-----e

The coronary artery that reaches the crux and supplies the posterior interventricular branch is termed the dominant coronary artery.the dominant coronary artery is usually the right coronary artery (85%).(CHAPTER 22,G)

16.----c

Fetal systemic arteries receives blood via the patent foramen ovale and PDA. (CHAPTER 23,G)

17.----d

PDA,APW,ASD and VSD are acyanotic conditions. (CHAPTER 23 ,G)

18.-----c

Rounding of the cardiac apex may suggest left ventricular hypertrophy. (CHAPTER 24 ,.G)

19.-----b (CHAPTER 24 ,G)

20.----a (Chapter 19,G)

21.----c

A nodular pattern is a feature of both interstitial disease and airspace disease. (Chapter 19, G)

22.----b

Air bronchograms and pseudocavitation may be particularly seen in bronchiolo-alveolar carcinoma and adenocarcinoma. .(Chapter 18,G)

23.----d

Simple pneumonia rarely causes radiographically visible hilar adenopathy, though enlarged central nodes may be seen on CT or MRI. Lung abscess can occasionally be confused with bronchial carcinoma because it may result in hilar or mediastinal adenopathy. (Chapter 18,G)

24.----e

(Chapter 17, G)

25.----a

Occasionally the parenchyma and airways become filled with fluid owing to the presence of a central obstructing lesion with little or no associated volume loss, and the lobe may even be expanded giving rise to the appearance termed 'drowned lobe'(Chapter 17,G)

26.----d

Pulmonary vessels may appear increased in size and may be indistinct because of adjacent peribronchial inflammation fibrosis (Chapter 16, G)

27.---a

With complete rupture of a mainstem bronchus, the lung may sag to the floor of the pleural cavity—the 'fallen lung sign'—as the intact vessels are unable to support the lung.). (CHAPTER 20 ,G)

28.----c

Bronchial dilatation on CT is often manifested by visualization of bronchi within 1 cm of the costal pleura or abutting the mediastinal pleura. (Chapter 16, G)

29.-----d

Thymomas usually show homogeneous density and uniform enhancement after contrast medium. (G)

30.----d

The plain radiograph and CT features of thymic carcinoid are indistinguishable from those of thymoma. (G)

31.-----e

Exudative bilateral effusions are seen with metastatic disease, lymphoma, pulmonary embolism, rheumatoid disease, systemic lupus erythematosus (SLE), myxoedema rheumatoid disease, systemic lupus erythematosus (SLE), post-cardiac injury syndrome, myxoedema and some ascites-related effusions. (G)

32.-----a

Pleural fluid collects initially under the lung, As the amount of effusion increases, the posterior and then the lateral costophrenic angles become blunted, by which time a 200–500 ml effusion is present. It is unusual for it to remain localized in this site once its volume exceeds 200–300 ml. (G)

33.-----a (webb)

34.-----b (Webb)

35.-----a
The two most common types of complete vascular rings are double aortic arch and right aortic arch with left ligamentum arteriosum, which account for 85–95% of cases. (CHAPTER 27 – The Aorta, including Intervention,Adam: Grainger & Allison's Diagnostic Radiology, 5th ed)

36.----b
The association of silicosis and rheumatoid arthritis (Caplan's syndrome) is more common than systemic sclerosis (Erasmus syndrome). (Chapter 19, G)

37.---b
The most common manifestation of asbestos exposure is pleural plaques. (Chapter 19,G)

38.----a
(CHAPTER 23.G)

39.----a
(CHAPTER 23,G)

40.------e
Thallium is an excellent tracer of myocardial perfusion but has significant limitations. The long physical half-life results in a radiation dose of the same order as coronary angiography. The relatively low injected dose results in a low signal-to-noise ratio and images can be suboptimal, especially in obese patients. Third, the relatively low-energy emission leads to low-resolution images and significant attenuation by soft tissue. (CHAPTER 22,G)

41.----b

Imaging starts within 5-10 min of injection of thallium and should be completed within 30 min. (CHAPTER 22,G)

42.----d
When T1- and T2-weighted imaging sequences are combined with gradient-echo cine-based functional cardiac imaging, both pericardial disease and its impact on cardiac function can be assessed. (Chapter 14, G)

43.------c
Chest radiograph findings in complete absence of the left pericardium include displacement of the heart into the left chest and interposition of lung between the aorta and pulmonary artery, as well as between the left hemidiaphragm and cardiac silhouette. Both the medial and lateral borders of the main pulmonary artery may be visualized more clearly due to absence of the anterior pericardial reflection between the aorta and the pulmonary artery. (Chapter 14,G)

44.----a
Cardiac rupture is not a uncommon complication in myocardial infarction. (CHAPTER 25,G)

45.------e
Adequacy of arterial flow can be assessed with intravascular Doppler.(CHAPTER 25,G)

46.----d
(CHAPTER 6,G)

47.----a
(CHAPTER 24 ,G)

48.----d

A moderate contrast enhancement
is noted . (CHAPTER 24 ,G)

49.----a
(CHAPTER 24,G)

50.----c
(CHAPTER 24 .G)

TEST PAPER 7

1.True regarding imaging of thymus
a. In younger patients, the CT density of the thymus is heterogenous and close to that of other soft tissues
b. after puberty the CT density gradually increases
c. above 40 years of age the thymus usually has CT attenuation value identical to that of muscle
d.the intensity of the thymus in T1-weighted images is similar to that of muscle and appreciably higher than that of mediastinal fat
e.On T2-weighted images, the intensity differences between the mediastinal fat and thymus are slight and do not vary with age.

2.All are true regarding mediastinal lymph nodes except
a. Ninety-five per cent of normal mediastinal lymph nodes are less than 15 mm in diameter
b. Lymph nodes in the paraspinal areas, in the region of the brachiocephalic veins and in the space behind the diaphragmatic crura are generally 6 mm or less in size
c. size of nodes in the aortopulmonary window, pretracheal and lower paratracheal spaces, and subcarinal are often 6–10 mm in diameter.
d. Highest mediastinal nodes lie just above a horizontal line drawn tangential to the upper margin of the aortic arch
e. The AJCC–UICC classification of lymph nodes are based on cross-sectional imaging

3.All are causes of opacification of hemithorax except
a. Pleural effusion and cosolidation
b. emphsema
c. Collapse
d. Fibrothorax and Massive tumour
e. Pneumonectomy and Lung agenesis

4.All are features of pleural effusion in supine position except
a. the meniscus effect
b. a hazy opacity like a veil affecting the whole or the lower part of the hemithorax
c.thickening of the minor fissure and widening of the paraspinal interface.
d. haziness of the diaphragmatic margin,
e. a pleural cap to the lung apex

5.The most common extragonadal site of germ-cell tmour
a.neck
b.mediastinum
c.upper abdomen
d.lower abdomen
e.head

6.All are true regarding mature teratoma in mediastinum except
a.m/c germ cell tumour
b.mostly solid

c.may have fat

d.may have calcification

e.located in anterior mediastinum

7.All are true regarding staphylococcal bronchopneumonia except

a. scattered multifocal heterogeneous opacities

b. Pleural effusion / empyema/ cavitation common

c. air bronchograms unusual

d. Pneumatoceles ,particularly in children

e. unilateral distribution

8.All are true regarding anaerobic pneumonia except

a. appearance of pneumonia is usually delayed ,24–72 h in aspiration

b. nearly two-thirds of lung abscess occur in the apicoposterior segments of upper lobes and the superior segments of lower lobes

c. aspiration pneumonia is seen in dependent lung segments (posterior upper lobe, superior, or posterobasal lower lobe.)

d. uni- or bi-lateral involvement in aspiration pneumonia

e. Empyema always occur with radiographic evidence of pneumonia

9.The cardinal sign of bronchiectasis on CT is

a. lack of tapering of bronchial lumina

b. internal bronchial diameter less than that of the adjacent pulmonary artery

c. visualization of bronchi within 1 cm of the costal pleura

d. visualization of bronchi abutting the mediastinal pleura

e. mucus-filled dilated bronchi

10.Internal bronchial diameter greater than that of the adjacent pulmonary artery seen on HRCT of bronchiectsis case is known as

a. signet ring sign

b. water lily sign,

c.camalote sign

d. rising sun sign

e.serpent sign

11.Which investigation provide more accurate delineation of tumour from postobstructive collapsed lung

a.PET

b.CT

c.MRI

d.ultrasound

e.chest x ray

12.All are true regarding right upper lobe collapse except

a. increased density at the apex of the hemithorax adjacent to the right side of the mediastinum

b. the elevated horizontal fissure resulting in a convex inferior outline

c. simulate an apical cap of pleural fluid or mediastinal widening on the frontal radiograph

d. elevation and a more horizontal course of the lower lobe pulmonary artery and right main bronchus

e. a triangular density with the base anteriorly against the chest wall and the apex at the hilum on CT

13.All are true regarding bronchogenic carcinoma except

a. The cardinal imaging signs of a central tumour are collapse/consolidation of the lung beyond the tumour and the presence of hilar enlargement

b. Dense hilum may be the only indication of lung cancer on PA view

c. hilar or mediastinal lymphadenopathy are seen in small cell carcinoma and large cell carcinoma

d. A peripheral nodule is very common in adenocarcinoma (72% of cases) and large cell tumours (63% of cases)

e. Adenocarcinoma cavitate more frequently than the other cell types

14. All are true regarding bronchiole-alveolar carcinoma except

a. arise from the alveoli and the immediately adjacent small airways

b. a solitary lobulated or spiculated pulmonary mass---uncommon on x ray

c. may show Bubble-like lucencies

d. may appears an ill-defined opacity resembling as bronchopneumonia

e. a lepidic (scale-like) growth pattern or focal ground-glass opacity

15.All are true of nodules in HRCT except

a.preponderance of nodules in relation to the major fissures and perhilar peribronchovascular interstitium in sarcoidosis

b.preponderance of nodules in centrilobular and subpleural location in silicosis and CWP

c.lower lobe predominance in sarcoidosis

d.beaded septum in lymphangitic spread of carcinoma

e.micronodule refers to size no larger than 7mm in diameter (the Fleishner society)

16.All are correctly matched HRCT finding of idiopathic interstitial fibrosis except

a. Idiopathic pulmonary fibrosis---- reticular opacities and ground glass opacity

b. Non-specific interstitial pneumonia—prominent ground glass opacity

c. Cryptogenic organizing pneumonia---Perilobular pattern

d. Acute interstitial pneumonia--- Consolidation (dependent lung)

e. Respiratory bronchiolitis– interstitial lung disease (RB–ILD)--- Poorly defined centrilobular nodules

17.Thin-walled discrete cysts is feature of which idiopathic interstitial fibrosis

a. Idiopathic pulmonary fibrosis

b. Non-specific interstitial pneumonia

c. Cryptogenic organizing pneumonia

d. Acute interstitial pneumonia-

e. Lymphoid interstitial pneumonia (LIP)

18.All are true regarding traumatic aortic rupture except

a. In clinical series, 90% of aortic ruptures occur at the ascending aorta

b. Seventy per cent of all patients with aortic rupture die at the scene of trauma

c. Traumatic aortic rupture is the cause of 16% of motor vehicle accident deaths

d. Untreated survivors invariably develop a chronic pseudoaneurysm at the site of the tear

e. the ascending aorta ruptures are usually rapidly fatal

19.All are features of mediastinal haematoma in chest x-ray except

a. Widening of the mediastinum

b. Blurring of the contours of the aortic arch and filling in of the aortopulmonary window

c. A right apical pleural cap

d. Deviation of the trachea or a nasogastric tube to the right and depression of the left mainstem bronchus.

e. Widening of the right paratracheal stripe and the paraspinal lines

20.All are features of interstitial edema except

a. thickening of the interlobular septa

b. peribronchial cuffing

c. conspicuous central pulmonary vessels

d. thickening of the interlobar fissures

e. lamellar 'effusion' in the costophrenic recesses

21.All are true regarding alveolar edema except

a. sparing of the apices and extreme lung bases in general

b.bilateral opacification

c.'butterfly' or 'bat's wing' distribution

d. alveologram

e. lower lobe blood diversion

22.All are true regarding right atrium except

a. the crista terminalis separates the body of the atrium from the appendage

b. The broad-based, squat right atrial appendage characterizes the morphological right atrium

c. The fossa ovalis lies in the middle of the interatrial septum

d. The coronary sinus enters the posterior wall of the right atrium between the tricuspid valve and the superior vena cava

e. superior and inferior venae cavae enter the posterior wall of the right atrium

23.All are causes of enlarged right atrium except

a. VSD

b. Restrictive cardiomyopathy

c. carcinoid syndrome

d. Pulmonary hypertension

e. Sinus of Valsalva fistula

24.Central cyanosis may be present within a few hours after birth in

a. tetralogy of Fallot

b. uncorrected transposition of great arteries (UTGA).

c. common atria and common ventricles

d. PDA

e. persistent truncus arteriosus

25.Cause of plethora with cyanosis is

a. Anomalous pulmonary veins

b. Ostium primum defect

c. Ostium secundum defect

d. Muscular ventricular septal defect (VSD)[

e.Patent arterial duct

26.In stable patients, what is the most accurate method for delineating diseases of the thoracic aorta and simultaneous evaluation of the left ventricular function.

a.Echo

b.CMR

c.MDCT

d.PET

e.Chest x ray

27.The technique of choice for displaying cusp perforation and aortic root abscess

a. transoesophageal US

b.transthoracic US

c.MDCT

d.PET

e.Chest x ray

28.All are true regarding secondary pulmonary nodule except

a.smallest unit of lung tissue marginated by connective tissue septa

b.irregularly polyhedral in shape

c.each lobule supplied by small bronchiole and pulmonary artery

d.pulmonary vein and lymphatic branches in the centre of lobule

e.made up of usually a dozen or fewer pulmonary acini

29.All are true regarding echocardiography role in IHD except

a. Assess ventricular function

b. detecting structural complication

c. echo contrast medium donot enhance the accuracy of assessment of ventricular function

d. Stress echo is useful for risk stratification in patients with known or suspected IHD

e. Stress echo is used for risk stratification after myocardial infarction, pre-operative risk assessment and determining viability

30.All are true of role of echo except

a. The origins of the main coronary arteries can not be imaged in children

b. Excellent images of proximal coronary arteries can be obtained by transoesophageal echocardiography

c. Echocardiography is very useful in detecting coronary artery aneurysms in Kawasaki disease.

d. Exercise echocardiography, with a threshold for significant disease of 50%, has sensitivity of 71–97% with overall accuracy of 69–92%.

e.dobutamine echocardiography, with a threshold for significant disease of 50%, has sensitivity of 70–96% with overall accuracy of 76–92%

31.All are true regarding Kerley A lines except

a. approximately 4 cm in length
b.most conspicuous in the upper and mid portions of the lung.
c.deep septal lines (lymphatic channels) that radiate from the hila into the central portions of the lungs
d. do not reach the pleura.
e. normally indicates a less acute or less degree of oedema.

32.All of the following are true regarding septal lines and blood vessels except
a. Septal lines are not visible in the outer 1 cm of the lung.
b.deep septal lines do not branch uniformly
c.septal lines are seen with a greater clarity than blood vessel of similar caliber
d. septal lines may disappear after treatment
e. pneumoconiosis cause persistent septal lines

33.All are true regarding adult type of coarctation except
a. usually distal to the ductus arteriosus and the left subclavian artery
b. Rib notching usually takes several years to develop
c. a '3' sign
d. cardiomegally
e.superior rib notching

34.All are true regarding rib notching in coarctation of aorta except
a.inferior rib notching
b. always bilateral but asymmetric
c. most often spares the first two ribs
d. usually have a corticated margin

e.due to enlarged and tortuous intercostal arteries

35.All are true except
a. Massive haemoptysis is defined as more than 300 ml of blood loss over 24h
b. The bronchial arteries arise anterolaterally from the descending thoracic aorta at the level of the fifth or sixth thoracic vertebra
c. the most common configurations of bronchial artery are of an intercostobronchial trunk (ICBT) on the right and two bronchial arteries on the left
d. A descending thoracic aortogram can rapidly identify any hypertrophied bronchial arteries
e. Embolization is usually performed using coils

36.All are true regarding bronchial artery embolisation except
a. bronchial artery are catheterized selectively with cobra, sidewinder, or multipurpose catheters
b. Bronchial embolization provides immediate relief of symptoms in 25% of cases
c. The source of haemorrhage lies in the bronchial arteries in 85–90% and in non-bronchial arteries in 10–15% of cases
d. spinal cord ischaemia causing myelitis or paraplegia may be the complication
e. Embolization is usually performed using polyvinyl alcohol particles of 300–500µm

37.Effects of ventilation in respiratory syndrome
a. pneumothorax
b. pulmonary interstitial emphysema (PIE).
c. Bronchopulmonary dysplasia (BPD) or chronic lung disease of prematurity (CLD)
d. Wilson–Mikity syndrome
e.all

38.All are true except
a. increased sharpness of the mediastinal border extending from the superior extent of the lung to the diaphragm in pneumothorax
b. The thymus compression by the pneumothorax
c. small bubbles of air radiating out from the hilum noted in pulmonary interstitial emphysema (PIE)
d. high-frequency ventilation may improve PIE
e. patchy or linear strands of increased density with localized areas of unequal aeration and generalized hyperaeration noted in Bronchopulmonary dysplasia (BPD)

39. A male child of 5 years is suffering from persistent cough with green colored sputum. Increased ratios of residual volume to total lung capacity is noted in pulmonary function test. A Cl⁻ concentration of sweat >70 meq/L is noted on lab investigation.Which is not the expected chest X-ray /HRCT finding of this case
a.central bronchiectasis

b. pleural effusion
c.bronchial wall thickening
d.tree-in bud appearance
e.mucous plugging

40.A male child of 15 yrs is suffering from persistent cough with green colored sputum. Increased ratios of residual volume to total lung capacity is noted in pulmonary function test.A Cl⁻ concentration of sweat >70 meq/L is noted on lab investigation.All are early finding on chest x-ray /HRCT of this case except
a.hyperinflation+thickening of the wall of the right upper lobe bronchus+bronchiectasis
b. hyperinflation+thickening of the wall of the right upper lobe bronchus +tree-in bud appearance
c. hyperinflation +tree-in bud appearance+bronchiectasis
d. thickening of the wall of the right upper lobe bronchus +tree-in bud appearance +bronchiectasis
e.bronchiectasis + thickening of the wall of the right upper lobe bronchus +tree-in bud appearance

41.A sexually promiscuous male patient was suffering from fever of unknown origin and chronic cough .He was diagnosed with AIDS .Which is typical feature of pneumocystis carnii infection of lung?
a.diffuse bilateral interastitial /alveolar infiltrates or both
b.asymmetric or nodular infiltrates and military nodules

c.apical disease and cyst ,pneomothoraces
d.lobular pneumonia and adenopathy
e.cavitary nodules and effusions

42. All are true regarding PMF except

a. much more common in CWP than in silicosis
b. as mass-like opacities, typically in the posterior upper lobe
c. The outer margins of PMF often parallel the contour of the adjacent chest wall
d. the presence of lobar volume loss
e. peripheral emphysema

43.All are true regarding aortic aneurysm except

a. commonly atherosclerotic
b. Marfan's and Ehlers–Danlos -- most commonly affect the aortic root, ascending aorta and arch
c. Ninety-five per cent of atherosclerotic aneurysms affect the thoracic aorta
d. Matrix metalloproteinases (MMPs) play an important role in the remodelling process
e. The asymptomatic thoracic aortic aneurysm (TAA) is often detected as a soft tissue mediastinal mass

44.All are true regarding aortic aneurysm except

a. ultrasound is the imaging method of choice for abdominal aorta aneurysm
b. Curvilinear calcification noted in abdominal aortic aneurysm
c. may be anterior erosion of the vertebral bodies

d. an abdominal aortic aneurysm below 5.5 cm (not enlarging rapidly and asymptomatic) require intervention
e. MDCT has made the diagnosis and evaluation of the extent of an aneurysm easy

45.All are true regarding endovasculat treatment of aortic aneurysm except

a. left subclavian artery can be covered if both vertebral arteries are patent.
b. The incidence of paraplegia is much higher with thoracic stent grafts than with surgery
c. Length of the aneurysm neck from the lowest renal artery to the origin of the aneurysm should to be at least 15 mm.
d. conical necks may lead to poor proximal seals or late endoleaks
e. most AAA stent grafts are bifurcated

47.All are true except

a.Weibel axial fibre system comprises the peribronchial and intralobular interstitium
b.the diameters of vessels and their neighboring bronchi are approximately equal
c.outer walls of bronchi and pulmonary vessels are smooth and sharply defined
d.bronchi are usually invisible within the peripheral 2cm of lung
e. vessels are well seen within the peripheral 2cm of lung

48.All are true regarding pulmonary features of cystic fibrosis except

a.bronchiectasis

b., cavitation
c. pulmonary fibrosis
d. pulmonary hypertension
e. conical-shaped chest

49.All are true regarding distribution of honeycombing except

a. the honeycombing in IPF and asbestosis are most severe in the subpleural lung regions and at the lung bases
b. the honeycombing in chronic hypersensitivity pneumonitis tends to be most severe in the midlung field with relative sparing of lung bases.
c. honeycombing in sarcoidosis may have an upper lobe predominance
d.fibrosis following ARDS has posterior distribution
e.subpleural,posterior and lower lobe predominant honeycombing highly suggestive of UIP.

50.All are true of honeycombing except

a.indicate presence of end stage disease
b.the presence of small air-containig cystic spaces

c.clearly visible walls
d.subpleural honeycombing occur in single layer
e.often predominate in the peripheral and subpleural lung regions

TEST PAPER 7(ANSWER)

1.-----e
In younger patients, the CT density of the thymus is homogeneous and close to that of other soft tissues.After puberty the CT density gradually decreases owing to fatty replacement.above 40 years of age the thymus usually has CT attenuation value identical to that of fat.The intensity of the thymus in T1-weighted images is similar to that of muscle and appreciably lower than that of mediastinal fat. (G)

2.---- d
Highest mediastinal nodes lie above a horizontal line at the upper rim of the bracheocephalic (left innominate) . (G)

3.-----b
Emphysema causes increased translucency. (G)

4.-----a
In the supine patient, pleural fluid layers out posteriorly and the meniscus effect, present from front to back, is not appreciated because of the projection. **(G)**

5.----b
The most common extragonadal site of germ-cell tmour is mediastinum. **(G)**

6.----b
Mature teratoma in mediastinum is mostly cystic. (G)

7.----e
Bilateral distribution noted in staphylococcal bronchopneumonia. Septicaemic infections, as opposed to those acquired by aspiration, cause disseminated, poorly marginated, peripheral, multifocal, nodules which can cavitate. (Chapter 15,G)

8.---e
Empyema is a common complication and occur with or without radiographic evidence of pneumonia. Multiple cavities reflecting severe lung necrosis may be seen 1–3 weeks following aspiration. (Chapter 15, G)

9.---a
The cardinal sign of bronchiectasis on CT is lack of tapering of bronchial lumina (Chapter 16, G)

10.----a
Internal bronchial diameter greater than that of the adjacent pulmonary artery seen on HRCT of bronchiectsis case is known as signet ring sign. (Chapter 16,G)

11.----a
(Chapter 17, G)

12.----b
On the frontal radiographic view of a right upper lobe collapse, the collapsed lobe forms increased density at the apex of the hemithorax adjacent to the right side of the mediastinum, with the elevated horizontal fissure resulting in a concave inferior outline depending on the degree of collapse (Chapter 17,G)

13.---e
Squamous cell cancers cavitate

more frequently than the other cell types. (Chapter 18, G)

14.----b

The most common radiographic finding is a solitary lobulated or spiculated pulmonary mass indistinguishable from other types of carcinoma. (Chapter 18, G)

15.----c

Upper lobe predominance of nodules is seen in sarcoidosis.(Webb)

16.-----b

Non-specific interstitial pneumonia is characterized by areas of ground-glass opacity ± traction bronchiectasis and honeycombing minimal. (Chapter 19,G)

17.-----e

Lymphoid interstitial pneumonia (LIP) is characterized by areas of ground-glass opacity, centrilobular nodules, thickened interlobular septa, thin-walled discrete cysts. (Chapter 19, G)

18.---a

In clinical series, 90% of aortic ruptures occur at the isthmus, just distal to the origin of the left subclavian artery. Rapid deceleration at impact leads to shearing forces at the aortic isthmus, the junction between the relatively mobile arch and the descending thoracic aorta. Contributory factors include tethering by the ligamentum arteriosum and the 'osseous

pinch', which occurs between the anterior chest wall and the thoracic spine at impact. (CHAPTER 20 ,G)

19.----c

A left apical pleural cap due to extrapleural haematoma and possibly a left pleural effusion are features of mediastinal haematoma. . (CHAPTER 20,G)

20.-----c

A loss of conspicuity of the central pulmonary vessels (termed a perihilar haze) is a feature of interstitial edema. (CHAPTER 21 ,G)

21.----e

Redistribution of blood to the upper zones is seen in some patients with elevated pulmonary venous pressure .when this occurs, vessels in the upper zones appear larger than comparable vessels in the lower zones (this appearance is called upper lobe blood diversion). (CHAPTER 21,G)

22.------d

The coronary sinus enters the posterior wall of the right atrium between the tricuspid valve and the inferior vena cava. (CHAPTER 22,G)

23.----a (CHAPTER 22,G)

24.-----b

Central cyanosis may be present within a few hours after birth. This indicates a very severe abnormality, such as UTGA, in which the aorta arises from the right ventricle (ventriculo-arterial discordance) and thus conveys desaturated blood to the systemic circulation. Such an anomaly is not compatible with life unless there is shunting (ASD, VSD and PDA) which enables mixing of oxygenated and desaturated blood. Central cyanosis may develop within the next few months or years. Infants with tetralogy of Fallot usually develop this delayed cyanosis, due to an increasing degree of obstruction of the outflow of the right ventricle by muscle hypertrophy and fibro-elastosis. (CHAPTER 23 ,G)

25.----a
Most common causes of plethora with cyanosis are Anomalous pulmonary veins and common arterial trunk (persistent truncus arteriosus). (CHAPTER 23,G)

26.-----b (CHAPTER 24 ,G)

27.----a (CHAPTER 24 ,G)

28.—d
Secondary pulmonary lobule contain pulmonary vein and lymphatic branches in the connective tissue interlobular septa.(Webb)

29.---c
For patients who are poor echocardiography subjects, the use of echo contrast medium improves definition of the margins of the ventricular cavity and enhances the accuracy of echocardiography for assessing ventricular function. (CHAPTER 25,G)

30.----a
The origins of the main coronary arteries can usually be imaged by echocardiography in adults, and almost invariably in children, in the absence of thoracic deformity.(CHAPTER 25,G)

31.----e
Presence of Kerley A normally indicates a more acute or severe degree of oedema.(CHAPTER 26 ,G)

32.----a
Septal lines can be differentiated from blood vessels as the latter are not visible in the outer 1 cm of the lung. In addition, deep septal lines do not branch uniformly (as is the case for blood vessels) and are seen with a greater clarity (as they represent a sheet of tissue) than a blood vessel of similar calibre. Under normal circumstances septal lines caused by interstitial fluid overload would be expected to disappear after suitable reduction in pulmonary venous pressure.(CHAPTER 26 ,G)

33.----d
Rib notching is caused by pressure erosion of the inferior aspects of the upper adjacent ribs by enlarged and tortuous intercostal arteries. .(CHAPTER 27 – The Aorta, including Intervention,Adam: Grainger & Allison's Diagnostic Radiology, 5th ed)

34.-----b
Rib notching in coarctation of aorta is usually bilateral(not always) but asymmetric, and most often spares the first two ribs where intercostal arteries arise from the costocervical trunk proximal to the usual site of coarctation and do not form part of the collateral circulation.
Unilateral absence of rib notching

is seen—on the left in the presence of a stenosed or occluded left subclavian artery, and on the right in association with anomalous origin of the right subclavian artery from below the level of the coarctation. .(CHAPTER 27 ,G)

35.----e
Embolization is usually performed using polyvinyl alcohol particles of 300–500μm. Massive haemoptysis is defined as more than 300 ml of blood loss over 24h. Moderate haemoptysis is more than three episodes of 100 ml d⁻ within 1 week (CHAPTER 28 ,G)

36.-----b
Bronchial embolization provides immediate relief of symptoms in 75% of cases. If bleeding does not stop immediately, repeat angiography and embolization should be performed. The source of haemorrhage lies in the bronchial arteries in 85–90% and in non-bronchial arteries in 10–15% of cases. The pulmonary arteries are rarely the cause of massive haemoptysis. (CHAPTER 28,G)

37-----e
(CHAPTER 64,G)

38----d
high-frequency ventilation may reduce the incidence of pneumothorax but in some cases PIE may become worse due to further air trapping. **(CHAPTER 64 ,G)**

39.----b (Webb)

40.----b (Webb)

41.-----a
Others are atypical features of pneumocystis carnii (webb)

42-----a
PMF refers to the coalescence of large nodules and is much more common in silicosis than in CWP. (Chapter 19, G)

43-----c
Ninety-five per cent of atherosclerotic aneurysms affect the abdominal rather than the thoracic aorta. (CHAPTER 27,G)

44----d
An abdominal aortuc aneurysm below 5.5 cm (not enlarging rapidly and asymptomatic) regular follow-up MDCT only.(CHAPTER 27 ,G)

46.----b
a large radicular artery supplying the spinal cord could be covered by a stent graft. The incidence of paraplegia is much lower with thoracic stent grafts than with surgery but is still 2% and can be devastating. .(CHAPTER 27,G)

47.----a
Weibel axial fibre system comprises the peribronchial and centrilobular interstium.The subpleural interstitium and interlobular septa are parts of the peripheral fibre system of Weibel.The intralobular interstitium bridges the gap between the centrilobular interstitium and interlobular septa

and subpleural interstitium.Bronchi less than 2mm in diameter are not normally visible on HRCT.

48.----e (Webb)

49.---d

Fibrosis following ARDS has anterior distribution(Webb)

50.----d

Subpleural honeycomb cysts occur in several contiguous layers.In paraseptal emphysema,subpleural cysts occur in a single layer (Webb).

TEST PAPER 8

1. A sexually promiscuous male patient was suffering from fever of unknown origin and chronic cough .He was diagnosed with AIDS.Sputum smear for AFB is negative .CD$_4$ count was less than 200 per mm^3.The pattern of TB in HIV+ patients differs from non-AIDS patients .The finding more frequently seen in such patients is/are all except

a. cavitation

b.resamble primary TB

c.mediastinal adenopathy

d.miliary disease

e.atypical infiltrates

2.A sexually promiscuous male patient was suffering from fever of unknown origin and chronic cough .He was diagnosed with AIDS.Sputum smear for AFB is negative .CD$_4$ count was less than 200per mm^3.The pattern of TB in HIV+ patients differs from non-AIDS patients.CT findings less common in HIV –postive patients are all except

a.cavitation

b.miliary spread

c.endobronchial spread

d.nodules 10-30mm and bronchial wall thickening

e.cosolidation

3.A middle aged immunocompetent female patient was suffering from chronic cough and hemoptysis but no fever All features are found in atypical nontuberculous mycobacterial infections except

a.bronchiectasis

b.small nodules

c.tree-in-bud

d.lower lobe predominance

e.consolidation

4.All are true regarding bronchopulmonary dysplasia except

a. the number of babies affected by BPD has increased

b. oxygen dependency at 28 days of age

c. patchy or linear strands of increased density

d. localized areas of unequal aeration

e. generalized hypo-aeration

5.Features of Wilson–Mikity syndrome are all except

a. in immature infants who are initially well

b.signs of respiratory distress in the second week

c. The lungs develop streaky

opacification and small cystic lucencies throughout lung

d. Respiratory failure ----may be progressive

e.all

6.All are true regarding carotid artery except

a. Selective carotid angiography is associated with a risk of stroke in 10 % of procedures

b. the sidewinder may be used in carotid angiography

c. the diagnosis of ICA stenosis is generally made noninvasively by duplex ultrasound, CTA, or MRA

d. ECST and NASCET trials showed benefit in surgically treating patients with 70–99% stenosis.

e.The criteria for treating patients with angioplasty and stenting are the same as for surgery

7.Lower limb vein thrombosis or oedema due to a common iliac occlusive lesion is referred to as

a. Paget–Schroetter syndrome

b. May–Thurner syndrome

c.Mary-John syndrome

d.Breslow syndrome

e.Patau syndrome

8.The imaging technique of choice in both infantile and adult coarctation of aorta

a.chest xray

b.CT

c.MRI

d.USG

e.PET

9.All are true regarding management of coarctation of aorta except

a. PTA is the primary method of treatment in adults, adolescents and children outside of infancy

b. resection and end-to-end anastomosis gives the best long-term result

c. the most usual procedure is repair by subclavian patch on failure of resection and anastomosis

d. Synthetic graft material is ideal in children

e. PTA success is defined as a reduction in gradient across a coarctation to less than 20 mmHg

10.All are true regarding except

a. '3' sign seen in pseudo coarctation

b. Aortic atresia is associated with hypoplastic left heart syndrome

c. Interrupted aortic arch is almost always associated with a large VSD

d. Type B Interrupted aortic arch refers to distal to the left common carotid artery

e. Patients with type A Interrupted aortic arch often have the DiGeorge syndrome

11.All are causes of persistent septal lines except

a. in long-standing PVH

b.idiopathic interstitial fibrosis

c.lymphangitis carcinomatosa

d. pneumoconiosis

e.pulmonary edema

12. Perihilar bat's wing' pattern of airspace consolidation is seen in

a.left ventricular failure

b.renal failure

c. a+b

d.cardiomyopathy

e.a+b+c

13.All are desirable characteristics of prosthetic cardiac valves except

a. lasting structural durability

b.capable of successful implantation in the native valve annulus

c.chemically inert

d.free of thrombogenicity,

e. offer abundant resistance to blood flow

14.All are complications of prosthetic cardiac valves except

a. paravalvar leak

b. occluder variance/erosion

c. strut fracture

d True aneurysm

e. post-pericardiotomy syndrome

15.All are causes of oligaemia except

a.Ebstein's anomaly

b.Tetralogy of Fallot

c. Uncorrected transposition of the great arteries with atrial or venous septal defect

d. Uhl's disease

e. persistent truncus --Type IV

16.All are causes of pulmonary edema except

a. Total anomalous pulmonary venous drainage

b. Fibro-elastosis of left ventricle

c. Cardiomyopathy

d. Coarctation of aorta

e. Tetralogy of Fallot

17.All are true regarding right ventricle except

a. a muscular conus or infundibulum separates the pulmonary valve from the tricuspid valve

b. coarsely trabeculated apex

c. the parietal band

d. no contribution to the cardiac silhouette in the frontal projection

e. the crista supraventricularis located at the upper end of septal aspect of conus.

18.The most common cause of a right ventricle enlargement

a.left heart failure

b. cor pulmonale

c. Chronic thromboembolic disease

d. Left-to-right shunt

e. Idiopathic pulmonary hypertension

19.All are true regarding pulmonary edema except

a. upper lobe blood diversion in cardiogenic pulmonary edema

b. A peripheral distribution of odema in ARDS

c. pleural effusions in cardiogenic edema

d.vascular pedicle width increased in cardiogenic edema

e.interstitial fluid in ARDS

20.Diffuse pulmonary haemorrhage is noted in all except

a.Marfan syndrome

b. Systemic lupus erythematosus

c. Wegener's granulomatosis

d. Fibrillary glomerulonephritis

e. Antibasement membrane antibody disease

21.All are true regarding aspiration except

a. Radiographic infiltrates normally appear within a few hours of aspiration of gastric contents

b. often progress for 24–48 h and most cases show evidence of regression after 72 h

c. more pronounced radiological abnormality noted on aspiration of acidic gastric contents

d. usually bilateral or mainly right sided

e. most commonly seen in the bases or superior segments of the lower lobes

22.All are features of cardiogenic pulmonary edema except

a. enlarged vascular pedicle

b. Upper lobe blood diversion

c. interstitial lines (Kerley A and B lines) and peribronchial cuffing

d. Pleural effusions

e. Patchy, peripheral air space opacification

23.All are true regarding usual interstitial pneumonia (UIP) except

a. areas of fibrosis at different stages of maturity

b. upper lobe irregularities (reticulation)

c. predominantly subpleural bibasal reticular pattern

d. honeycombing

e. ground-glass opacification a dominant feature

24.The rapid development of a diffuse increase in the attenuation of lung parenchyma in patients with IPF raise the possibility

a. an opportunistic infection (such as PCP)

b. an accelerated phase of the

disease

c. concurrent pulmonary oedema

d. a+b

e.a+b+c

25.All are criteria for T2 tumour of bronchogenic tumour except

a. A tumour less than 3 cm in its greatest dimension

b. tumour of any size that invades the visceral pleura

c. a tumour of any size that has associated atelectasis or obstructive pneumonitis extending to the hilar region

d. the proximal extent of demonstrable tumour within a lobar bronchus at bronchoscopy

e. the proximal extent of demonstrable tumour at least 2 cm distal to the carina at bronchoscopy

26.T3 bronchogenic tumour extend to all except

a. chest wall

b.diaphragm

c. the mediastinal pleura

d. pericardium

e. heart

27.All are true regarding left upper lobe collapse except

a. veil-like' increased density of the whole of the affected hemithorax in most cases

b. loss of the normal silhouette of structures adjacent to the collapse(the left heart border, mediastinum, and aortic arch)

c. visibility of the aortic knuckle outline in less severe cases

d. increased angulation between the left main bronchus and the lower lobe bronchus

e. The Luftsichel sign(an 'air crescent' seen between the aortic arch and the medial border of the collapse)

28. Middle lobe syndrome refers to middle lobe of right lung with
a.collapse
b. broncheictasis
c. previous pulmonary tuberculosis
d. focal bronchostenosis
e.consolidation

29.All are features of HRCT of bronchiectasis except
a. serpent sign in varicose variety
b. beaded configuration of bronchi
c. a string of cysts/cluster of cysts
d. Air–fluid levels
e. lobulated gloved finger, V- or Y-shaped densities

30.All are true regarding bronchiectasis except
a. associated CT findings of bronchiolitis are seen in about 30% of patients with bronchiectasis
b. Small centrilobular nodular and linear branching opacities (tree-in-bud sign) express inflammatory and infectious bronchiolitis
c. MDCT with thin collimation is the technique of choice for the detection and the assessment of the extent of bronchiectasis.
d. Bilateral upper lobe distribution is most common in patients with cystic fibrosis and allergic bronchopulmonary aspergillosis

e. unilateral upper lobe distribution is most common in patients with tuberculosis

31.All are true regarding pneumonia except
a. The most common pattern in*Mycoplasma pneumoniae* is unilateral lower lobe involvement
b. Varicella causes pneumonia more frequently in children than in adult
c. Varicella shows widespread 5–10 mm in diameter poorly marginated nodules or acinar opacities
d. The nodules in varicella usually resolve in a week or two but can persist for months (simulating metastases)
e. numerous small irregular calcified nodules can be seen in varicella on reolution

32.All are true regarding primary tuberculosis except
a. involvement of any lobe
b. homogeneous pneumonia
c. Multifocal involvement unusual
d. cavitation rare
e. nodal enlargement, usually bilateral, hilar and/or mediastinal

33.All are true regarding malignant mediastinal tumour except
a. seen in young adults
b.> 90% cases in female
c. fat density not seen and visible calcification rare
d.secrete human chorionic gonadotrophin and α-fetoprotein
e.seminoma is most common variety

34. All are true regarding mediastinal lymphnode calcification except
a. common following tuberculosis and fungal infection
b. common in metastatic neoplasm
c. may be seen in lymph node metastases osteosarcoma, chondrosarcoma
d. foamy appearance seen with *Pneumocystis jiroveci* infection in AIDS patients
e. eggshell calcification in sarcoidosis

35. All are indication of CABG surgery or PCI except
a. severe CAD and angina which is not responding to medical treatment
b. unstable angina
c. severe left main coronary artery stenosis
d. angina persisting after myocardial infarction
e. positive stress test and severe disease of the corresponding coronary arteries

36. Low attenuation mediastinal nodes are seen in
a. tuberculosis
b. fungal diseases
c. metastases from testicular tumour
d. lymphoma
e. all

37. Mediatinal lymph node with CT number less than water is seen in
a. Wipples disease
b. tuberculosis
c. fungal diseases
d. metastases from testicular tumour
e. lymphoma

38. All are true regarding role of imaging in pleural effusion except
a. Ultrasound can be used to identify small amounts of pleural fluid,
b. The fat-containing chylothorax have a lower CT number than normal,
c. CT numbers do not allow a distinction between transudate and exudates
d. MRI may differentiate transudates from exudates using triple echo-pulse sequence
e. Chylous effusion causes high signal intensity on T1-weighted images

39. The most common cause of haemothorax is
a. trauma
b. ruptured aortic aneurysm
c. pneumothorax
d. extramedullary haemopoiesis
e. coagulopathies.

40. All are true regarding AJCC–UICC classification of regional lymph nodes except
a. Station 1 through 9 nodes lie within the mediastinal pleural envelope, whereas station 10 through 14 nodes lie outside the mediastinal pleura within the visceral pleura.
b. Subaortic (aortopulmonary window) nodes lie lateral to the ligamentum arteriosum
c. Highest mediastinal nodes lie above a horizontal line at the upper rim of the bracheocephalic (left innominate) vein
d. Hilar nodes lie distal to the mediastinal pleura reflection and

the nodes adjacent to the bronchus intermedius on the right
e. right and left lower paratracheal lymph node is referred as (stations 2R and 2L)

41.All true regarding junction lines in chest x ray except
a.the anterior junction line starts below the clavicles and continues well below the aortic arch.
b. the supra-aortic posterior junction line goes well above the level of the clavicles and extends down to the top of the aortic arch
c.the posterior junction line separates to envelop the aortic arch.
d. posterior junction line extends to the level of the lung apices
e. the lack of visualization of junctional areas is a reliable sign of mass in the junctional areas

42.All are true regarding mosaic perfusion except
a.due to regional decrease in lung perfusion
b.seen in bronchiolitis obliterans
c.vessels in involved area equal in size to that of uninvolved area
d.air trapping in case of airway disease
e.area of low attenuation are usually larger then lobules in vascular disease

43.All are true regarding earliest radiographic changes of silicosis except
a. profusion of small (1–3 mm) round nodules
b. distributed in the posterior

aspects of the upper two-thirds of the lung
c. nearly identical to the earliest radiographic changes and CWP
d. nodules in silicosis are often larger than CWP
e.eggshell calcification

44.HRCT of a patients shows mixed densities of mosaic perfusion,normal lung and ground-glass opacity .This is known as
a.Mixure sign
b.the Head-Cheese sign
c.halo sign
d.crazy-paving
e.Romana sign

45.Perilymphatic distribution of nodules are seen in all except
a.sarcoidosis
b.tuberculosis
c.silicosis
d.CWP
e.lymphangitic spread of carcinoma

46.The CT signs of diaphragmatic rupture are all except
a.discontinuity of the diaphragm
b.dependent viscera sign
c.thick crus sign
d.collar sign
e.Double –diaphragm sign

47.All are true regarding pericardium except
a. the 20–60-ml of pericardial cavity

b. the visceral pericardium extends the ascending aorta to a point 20–30 mm above the aortic root

c. The arterial mesocardium is higher on the right than left

d. the venous mesocardium has the shape of U

e. The arterial and venous mesocardia are connected by the transverse sinus

48.All are true regarding normal pericardium except

a. the normal pericardium seen as a 1–2-mm thick curved stripe anterior to the heart on lateral chest x-ray

b. The visceral pericardium is visualized separately by MRI

c. The combination of the visceral pericardium and the small layer of physiological pericardial fluid constitutes the normal pericardium

d. the pericardium is readily visualized overlying the right atrium and right ventricle in most individuals

e. pericardium is often not visible over the lateral and inferior walls of the left ventricle.

49.Continuous diaphragm sign is seen in

a. Mediastinal haemorrhage

b. Mediastinal emphysema

c. Fibrosing mediastinitis

d.diaphragmatic hernia

e.pericardial effusion

50.Coalmine dust and silica predispose workers to all except

a. chronic bronchitis

b.simple pneumoconiosis

c. emphysema

d.complicated pneumoconiosis (progressive massive fibrosis [PMF])

e.mesothelioma

TEST PAPER 8(ANSWER)

1-----**a** (Webb)

2-----**b** (Webb)

3-----**d**

Lingula and middle lobe predominance of lesion is noted in atypical nontuberculous mycobacterial infections.(Webb)

4.----**e**

Characteristic radiographic appearances of BPD are patchy or linear strands of increased density with localized areas of unequal aeration and generalized hyperaeration. **(CHAPTER 64,G)**

5-----**e (CHAPTER 64,G)**

6.-----**a**

Selective carotid angiography is associated with a risk of stroke in 1% of procedures. the sidewinder, the Berenstein, the Headhunter, or the Mani catheter may be used in carotid angiography.(CHAPTER 28 ,G)

7.-----**b**

Thoracic outlet syndrome is also known as Paget–Schroetter syndrome. Paget–Schroetter syndrome refers to acute subclavian or axillary vein thrombosis caused by underlying venous obstruction due to the muscles or bony structures of the thoracic outlet (CHAPTER 28 ,G)

8-----**c** (CHAPTER 27 ,G)

9.----**d**

Synthetic graft material is unsuitable in children because it does not stretch. (CHAPTER 27 ,G)

10----**e**

Interrupted aortic arch can occur distal to the left subclavian artery (type A, 30–40%), distal to the left common carotid artery (type B, 53%), or distal to the innominate artery (type C, 4%). Patients with type B often have a chromosomal abnormality called the DiGeorge syndrome. (CHAPTER 27,G)

11.----**e**

(CHAPTER 26 ,G)

12-----**c** (CHAPTER 6 ,G)

13----**e**

Prosthetic cardiac valves should offer little resistance to flow. (CHAPTER 24,G)

14.-----**d**

Pseudoaneurysm is a complication of prosthetic cardiac valve. Prosthetic cardiac valves should offer little resistance to flow. (CHAPTER 24 ,G)

15----**c**

Uncorrected transposition of the great arteries with atrial or venous septal defect produce plethora. (CHAPTER 23 ,G)

16----**e** (CHAPTER 23 ,G)

17----**e**

The lower end of the septal aspect of the conus has a discrete muscular elevation, the crista supraventricularis, extending to the right and forwards over the tricuspid valve to the right ventricular free wall to form the parietal band. .(CHAPTER 22 ,G)

18.---e (CHAPTER 22,G)

19----e
Interstitial edema is noted in cardiogenic edema. One of the classical radiographic manifestations of interstitial oedema is thickening of the interlobular septa. (CHAPTER 21 ,G)

20----a
Rheumatoid arthritis, Systemic sclerosis, Systemic necrotizing vasculitis, Microscopic polyarteritis, Rapidly progressive glomerulonephritis without immune complexes are other causes of Diffuse pulmonary haemorrhage. (CHAPTER 21,G)

21.---c
More pronounced radiological abnormality is noted when acidic gastric contents are aspirated. (CHAPTER 20,G)

22-----e
Cardiogenic pulmonary edema causes diffuse perihilar air space opacification. (CHAPTER 20.G)

23----e
The presence of ground-glass opacification is not a dominant feature. As the disease progresses, it often appears to 'creep' around the periphery of the lung to involve the anterior aspects of the upper lobes.(Chapter 19, G)

24----e
(Chapter 19, G)

25----a
Size of T2 tumour of bronchogenic tumour is more than 3 cm in its greatest dimension. (Chapter 18,G)

26----e
T3 tumour ------A tumour of any size with direct extension into the chest wall (including superior sulcus tumours), diaphragm, or the mediastinal pleura or pericardium without involving the heart, great vessels, trachea, oesophagus, or vertebral body; or a tumour in the main bronchus within 2 cm of the carina without involving the carina. (Chapter 18,G)

27----c
Paradoxically the aortic knuckle outline is visible in more severe cases as the apical segment of the left lower lobe is hyperexpanded superiorly adjacent to the aortic arch . (Chapter 17, G)

28----e
(Chapter 17,G)

29----a
Serpent sign is seen in hydatid cyst of lung. . (Chapter 16, G)

30----a
Associated CT findings of bronchiolitis are seen in about 70% of patients with bronchiectasis. . (Chapter 16,G)

31----b
Varicella is unlike other viruses in that it causes pneumonia more frequently in adults than in children. (Chapter 15, G)

32----e

Compared with community-acquired pneumonia, primary tuberculosis may exhibit nodal enlargement, usually ipsilateral, hilar and/or mediastinal. In fact, lymphadenopathy is the most common manifestation of primary tuberculosis in children and occurs with or without pneumonia (Chapter 15,G)

33----b

Malignant germ-cell tumours are usually seen in young adults and are much more common in men (>90%) than women. Seminoma is the most common form. Malignant germ-cell tumours secrete human chorionic gonadotrophin and α-fetoprotein, which can be used as markers to diagnose and monitor the tumour. (G)

34----b.

Mediastinal lymphnode calcification may be seen in lymph node metastases from calcifying primary malignancies, such as osteosarcoma, chondrosarcoma and mucinous colorectal and ovarian tumours, lymph node calcification is rare in metastatic neoplasm. It is virtually unknown in untreated lymphoma . (G)

35----b (CHAPTER 25,G)

36----e

(Chapter 14,**G**)

37----a

Attenuation values below that of water are seen in fatty replacement of inflammatory nodes and have also been described in Whipple's disease. (Chapter 14,G)

38---b

The fat-containing chylothorax does not have a lower CT number than normal, because of its protein content. **(G)**

39----a

The most common cause of haemothorax is trauma. (G)

40-----e

Right and left lower paratracheal is referred as (stations 4R and 4L) while right, left and posterior upper paratracheal is referred as (stations 2R, 2L) **(G)**

41----e

Since both junction lines are inconsistently seen, the lack of visualization of junctional line is not a reliable sign of disease. (G)

42-----c

Regardless of cause ,vessels in involved area (decreased opacity) often appear smaller than vessels in relatively dense areas of lung .(Webb)

43------e (Chapter 19,G)

44----b

Mixed densities of mosaic perfusion, normal lung and ground-glass opacity on HRCT is called the Head-Cheese sign because its remenblance to the variegated appearance of a sausage made from parts of the head of a hog.This sign is usually indicative of mixed infiltrative and obstructive disease,usually associated with bronchiolitis.(Webb)

45-----b(Webb)

46-----e

The CT signs of diaphragmatic rupture are discontinuity of the diaphragm with direct visualization of the diaphragmatic injury,herniation of abdominal organs with liver, bowel or stomach in contact with the posterior ribs ('dependent viscera sign'),thickening of the crus ('thick crus sign'),constriction of the stomach or bowel ('collar sign'), active arterial extravasation of contrast material near the diaphragm; and, in the case of a penetrating diaphragmatic injury, depiction of a missile or puncturing instrument trajectory. (G)

47-----d

The venous mesocardium has the shape of inverted U. Beneath the apex of the U is the space between the pulmonary veins and the left atrium --the oblique sinus. (Chapter 14, G)

48-----b

The visceral pericardium is normally very thin and is therefore not visualized separately by any imaging modality. The combination of the visceral pericardium and the small layer of physiological pericardial fluid constitutes the normal pericardium routinely visualized on CT and MRI as a 1–2-mm thick layer. (Chapter 14, The Mediastinum, Including the Pericardium, Adam: Grainger & Allison's Diagnostic Radiology, 5th ed)

49-----b

In Mediastinal emphysema ,air may track extraserosally on either side of the diaphragm, which is occaisionally seen as a continuous line of transradiancy known as the 'continuous diaphragm sign'. (Chapter 14, G)

50----e

Both coalmine dust and silica predispose workers to chronic bronchitis, simple pneumoconiosis, emphysema, complicated pneumoconiosis (progressive massive fibrosis [PMF]), lung cancer (in excess of that expected from smoking alone) and mycobacterial pulmonary infection—the risk for tuberculosis is increased three-fold in patients with chronic silicosis. (Chapter 19, G)

TEST PAPER 9

1.All are regarding right paratracheal stripe in chest x-ray except
a.consists of the right wall of the trachea and the adjacent mediastinal fat
b. visible stripe of uniform thickness
c.between the tracheal air column and the lung.
d. no more than 10 mm wide,
e. visible in approximately two-thirds of normal people.

2.All are true regarding azygo-esophageal line except
a. normally above azygos arch
b.traced down to posterior costophrenic angle in normal subjects
c. The upper few centimetres always straight or concave toward the lung
d.a convex shape suggests the presence of a subcarinal mass
e.a convex shape suggests the presence of left atrial enlargement

3.All are true regarding Primary spontaneous pneumothorax except
a.no obvious precipitating event and essentially normal lung
b. occurs predominantly in young adults
c. five times more common in men than women.
d. nearly always caused by the rupture of an apical pleural bleb

e. recurrence common in untreated case but on the contralateral side

4.All are spontaneous ,secondary causes of adult pneumothorax
a. Histiocytosis X
b. Lymphangioleiomyomatosis
c. Fibrosing alveolitis
d. Metastatic sarcoma
e.ILD

5. A low-density centre with rim enhancement of the enlarged mediastnal node is a useful pointer towards the diagnosis of
a.Wipples disease
b.tuberculosis
c.metastases from melanoma
d.metastases from testicular tumour
e.lymphoma

6.Strikingly uniform contrast enhancement of mediastinal lymph node enlargement is seen in
a.Wipples disease
b.tuberculosis
c.sarcoidosis
d. Castleman's disease
e.lymphoma

7.The most common manifestation of primary tuberculosis in children
a. hilar and/or mediastinal lymphadenopathy
b. pneumonia
c. Pleural effusion
d. segmental or lobar collapse
e. bronchopneumonia

8.All are true regarding pleural effusion in primary tuberculosis except
a. in children associated with parenchymal or nodal disease
b. frequently isolated in teenagers and young adults
c. pleural thickening and calcification
d. Residual pleural change is unusual
e. often large and unilateral

9.All are true regarding of chest findigs in cystic fibrosis except
a. Hyperinflation in early or mild disease
b. accentuated linear opacities in the upper lung areas
c. proximal bronchiectasis and mucoid impaction
d. cystic regions of the upper lobes
e. HRCT is not useful in asymptomatic patients

10.All are true regarding acute stage of allergic bronchopulmonary aspergillosis
a. transient consolidation,
b.atelectasis
c. a tendency of atelectasis to recur in the different area
d. Bronchoceles appearing as opacities of a variety of shapes
e. a recurrence of consolidation in the same area

11.All are true regarding lower lobe collapse except
a. displacement of oblique fissure posteriorly and medially
b. the collapsed lobe lies in the posteromedial portion of the chest
c. the collapsed lower lobes usually form a triangular density behind the heart on PA chest

d. The medial portion of the hemidiaphragm may be obscured
e. the vertebral column appears progressively less denser inferiorly

12.All are true regarding lower lobe collapse except
a. the lower lobe pulmonary artery is usually not seen in lower lobe collapse
b. The major airways, including the right and left main bronchi displaced more vertically in lower lobe collapse
c. the 'superior triangle sign' in left lower lobe collapse
d. The 'flat waist sign' in extensive collapse of the left lower lobe
e. loss of the outline of the superior aortic knuckle in severe left lower lobe collapse

13.N3 tumour involve all except
a. contralateral mediastinal lymph nodes
b.contralateral hilar lymph nodes
c.ipsilateral or contralateral scalene lymph nodes
d ipsilateral or contralateral supraclavicular lymph nodes
e.contralateral carinal lymph node

14.Very high likelihood of technical respectability of bronchogenic carcinoma if
a.tumour show less than 5cm of contact with mediastinum
b. tumour show less than 6cm of contact with mediastinum
c. tumour show less than 3cm of contact with mediastinum
d. tumour show less than 2cm of contact with mediastinum

e. tumour show less than 4cm of contact with mediastinum

15. Very high likelihood of technical respectability of bronchogenic carcinoma if

a.tumour shows less than 60 degrees of circumferential contact with the aorta

b.tumour shows less than 70 degrees of circumferential contact with the aorta

c.tumour shows less than 80 degrees of circumferential contact with the aorta

d.tumour shows less than 50 degrees of circumferential contact with the aorta

e.tumour shows less than 90 degrees of circumferential contact with the aorta

16.Non-specific interstitial pneumonia is characterized by all except

a. predominant pattern of ground-glass opacification

b. predominantly basal and subpleural distribution

c.fibrosis usually of uniform temporality

d. honeycombing

e. finer reticular pattern

17.All are true regarding diffuse pleural thickening except

a. dose related

b. results from thickening and fibrosis of the visceral pleura

c.cause of impairement lung function

d. CT is more sensitive and specific than chest radiography in the detection of diffuse pleural thickening

e. The frequency of diffuse pleural thickening increases with time from first exposure

18.All are true regarding cryptogenic organizing pneumonia except

a. Peripheral or peribronchial consolidation

b. more frequently in the upper zones

c. change of location of consolidation over time

d. perilobular pattern

e. The lung architecture and volume generally well preserved

19.All are true of pulmonary edema except

a. cardiac failure and overhydration are most common causes of pulmonary edema in ICU

b. Overhydration causes a more central distribution of oedema and a wider vascular pedicle compared with cardiogenic oedema

c. Central perihilar air space opacification is noted in renal cause of pulmonary edema

d. Pleural effusions is common in ARDS

e.Cardiomegaly noted in cardiogenic pulmonary edema

20.The preferred technique for confirming or excluding the presence of pulmonary embolism

in the ICU patient
a.chest xray
b. ventilation perfusion scintigraphy
c. catheter pulmonary angiography
d. CT pulmonary angiography (CTPA)
e.MR agngiography

21.'A reversed mismatch' on V/Q scan is noted in all except
a. lobar collapse
b. pneumonic consolidation
c. large pleural effusion
d. obstructive airway disease
e.non infarct causing pulmonary embolism

22.All are true regarding wegner's granulomatosis except
a. multiple nodules(few millimeters to several centimeters in diameter)
b. a feeding vessel leading to the nodule on CT
c. air bronchograms within lung nodules
d. Consolidation and ground-glass opacities
e. cavitation an invariable feature

23.All are true regarding cryptogenic organizing pneumonia except
a. Bilateral patchy areas of consolidation
b. no zonal predilection of lesions
c. propensity of consolidation for central regions
d.the 'reverse halo' sign
e. Nodules

24.All are true regarding left atrial appendage except

a. The left atrium usually receives the four pulmonary veins at the 'corners' of its anterior surface
b. The long finger-like forward-projecting left atrial appendage is its only characteristic morphological feature
c. the normal left atrial appendage is buried in the epicardial fat
d. The left atrium makes no definite contribution to the normal cardiac silhouette in the frontal view
e. In the lateral view the left atrium contributes to the upper posterior border of the heart

25.All are causes of left atrial enlargement except
a. Mitral regurgitation
b. Ventricular septal defect
c. Patent ductus arteriosus
d. Mitral stenosis
e. Anomalous pulmonary venous drainage

26.The features that best characterizes left ventricular morphology is
a. conical shape
b.relatively fine trabeculation (absent on the upper septum)
c. fibrous continuity of the entry atrioventricular valve and the exit semilunar valve
d. conus
e.infundibulum

27.All are true regarding pulmonary circulation except
a. enlarged central pulmonary arteries with smaller the peripheral pulmonary arteries in Eisenmenger reaction
b. Increased bronchial artery circulation in cyanotic CHD

c. pulmonary plethora recognized by enlarged central and peripheral pulmonary arteries and veins in all zones

d. Pulmonary venous congestion and oedema -- the result of the failure of the left heart

e. Tetralogy of Fallot shows plethora

28. Coeur en sabot is noted in

a.TOF

b.UCTGA

c. total superior anomalous pulmonary venous drainage

d. Ebstein's anomaly

e. Uhl's disease

29.All are central ball occluder valve except

a.Starr–Edwards

b. Smelloff–Cutter

c.Braunwald–Cutter

d. the Beall and Starr–Edwards 6500

e.Magovern–Cromie

30.All are correctly matched except

a. the Bjork–Shiley,Omniscience, and Medtronic–Hall --- Eccentric monocuspid disc valve

b. St Jude ,the Carbomedics and Sorin bicarbon valves---- Bileaflet disc valve

c. the Beall and Starr–Edwards 6500 series.----   Central caged disc occluder valve

d. the Starr–Edwards, Harken, Smelloff–Cutter---- Central ball occluder valve

e. Carpentier–Edwards ,the Hancock and the Ionescu–Shiley -- --mechanical valve

31.All are true regarding cardiac computed tomography and computed tomographic angiography except

a. partial rotation image reconstruction is helpful for cardiac CT

b.effective dose of coronary MDCTA is 6-8 mSv (constant tube current)

c. The value of CTA is well established in the evaluation of aortic disease

d. high calcification score (>400) strongly suggests a stenosis

e. MDCT doesnot accurately determine CABG patency

32.All are true regarding role of Cardiac magnetic resonance imaging and magnetic resonance angiography in IHD except

a.low signal on T2-weighted imaging in recent myocardial infarction

b.poor perfusion with first-pass contrast medium imaging in recent myocardial infarction

c.delayed enhancement with gadolinium-based perfusion agents in recent myocardial infarction

d.left ventricular dysfunction or aneurysm are well shown by cine-MRA and tagging sequences

e.DE-MRI is probably the best method for determining the size of the infarction in the acute myocardial infarction

33.Causes of noncardiogenic pulmonary edema is/are
a. Aspiration
b. Adult respiratory distress syndrome (ARDS)
c. Hepatorenal failure
d.Rapid lung re-expansion post thoracocentesis
e.All

34.All are correctly matched except
a. PCWP(8–12 mmHg) ----normal
b.PCWP (12–18 mmHg) ----upper lobe venous distension.
c.PCWP (19–25 mmHg) ----- interstitial oedema (peribronchial cuffing, Kerley lines).
d.PCWP > (25 mmHg) ----- airspace opacities
e.PCWP>40mmHg----airspace opacities

35.Causes of noncardiogenic pulmoray edema is /are
a. Aspiration
b. Adult respiratory distress syndrome (ARDS)
c. Hepatorenal failure
d. Rapid lung re-expansion post thoracocentesis
e.All

36.All are true regarding traumatic aortic injury except
a. incomplete rupture of the aorta noted in 80-90%
b.the most common site of injury(90%) ---the aortic isthmus
c. widening or abnormality of the mediastinum seen in 92.7% of patients
d. proposed upper limit of normal for mediastinal width (8 cm)
e. Thoracic aortography is accurate for diagnosis

37.Most commonly seen signs on chest x ray in case of traumatic aortic injury are all except
a. Irregularity or blurring of the aortic knuckle contour
b. Enlargement of the aortic knuckle
c. Downward displacement of left main stem bronchus
d. Upper mediastinal widening
e. Aortopulmonary window opacification

38.Indications of inferior vena cava filters are all except
a. to prevent fatal pulmonary embolism (PE) in patients with a documented PE
b. IVC, iliac or femoropopliteal DVT who cannot be treated with anticoagulants
c. protection against PE in pregnant women with proven DVT during caesarean section or childbirth
d. pre-operatively in patients with iliofemoral DVT when anticoagulation is contraindicated
e.all

39.All are true regarding inferior vena cava filters except
a. diameter of the IVC measured and the position of the renal veins documented
b. the ideal position for the IVC filter is in the infrarenal IVC with the apex of the filter at or just below the level of the renal veins
c. Filters can be inserted via the femoral or jugular venous route
d. ideal choice for retrieval is via

the femoral route

e. Suprarenal positioning of the filter in case of renal vein thrombosis

40----698.Bilateral pulmonary hypoplasia ,renal agenesis associated with oligohydramnios occurs in

a. Potter's syndrome

b. asphyxiating thoracic dystrophy

c. Wilson–Mikity syndrome

d. Paget–Schroetter syndrome

e. May–Thurner syndrome

41.All are true of meconium aspiration syndrome except

a. patchy areas of collapse

b. patchy areas of consolidation

c. hypoinflation in the peripheral lung

d. Pneumothorax and pneumomediastinum

e. persistent fetal circulation

42.Chest x ray of a young patient shows a solitary pulmonary nodule. On CT scan all are true except

a.homogenous and ring of calcification indicate of malignancy

b.Fat within SPN is diagnostic of hamartoma

c. pulmonary AVMshows enlarged feeding artery and draining vein

d. popcorn pattern of calcification noted in hamartoma

e.fat within consolidation indicate of lipoid pneumonia

43.Feeding vessel sign is noted on CT scan of chest in

a.hematogenous metastases

b.septic emboli

c.multiple pulmonary infarcts

d.Wegener's granulomatosis

e.all

44.All are predominantly upper lung disease except

a.sarcoidosis

b.LCH

c.cystic fibrosis

d.respiratory bronchiolitis

e.BOOP

45.Which drug toxicity mimic the pulmonary metastases and have histologic characteristic of BOOP

a.Busulphan

b.Methotrexate

c.Amiodarone

d.Bleomycin

e.Cyclophosphamide

46.Correctly matched findings are all except

a. Delayed hyperenhancement on contrast-enhanced MRI ---detect nonviable myocardium

b. Arrhythmogenic right ventricular dysplasia----focal thinning and abnormal motion of the right ventricle

c. Acute myocarditis: focal wall motion with abnormal high signal on T2-weighted images and contrast enhancement on T1-weighted images

d. sarcoidosis (high signal on T2-weighted images; contrast enhancement on T1-weighted or delayed contrast-enhanced MRI);

e. myocardial iron overload --- diffuse reduction in contraction, increased myocardial signal

47.All are true regarding Thallium 201 except

a. intravenously as thallous chloride

b. the usual dose is 80–110 mBq

c. 4% of the injected dose localizes in the myocardium

d. Distribution in the myocardium is proportional to perfusion

e. relatively short physical half-life

48.The most common congenital heart defect detected in adults

a.VSD

b.ASD

c.PDA

d.TAPVC

e.TOF

49.All are true regarding ventricular function except

a. The normal left ventricle ejects about two-thirds of its content with each beat, to produce an ejection fraction of 66%

b. In the resting state, localized contraction abnormalities usually represent areas of infarction

c. Significant overall impairment of the left ventricle is present if the ejection fraction falls below 50%

d. The severity of left ventricular dysfunction is one of the most important prognostic indicators of survival after myocardial infarction

e. Echo is probably the most accurate method for comprehensively assessing ventricular function

50.All are true regarding ASD except

a. Ostium secundum defects form about 80% of all ASDs

b. The ostium primum defect associated with partial anomalous pulmonary venous drainage.

c. risk factor for paradoxical thromboembolic stroke.

d. Transoesophageal echocardiography the main imaging technique used to assess ASDs

e. Ostium secundum defects are located in the fossa ovalis

TEST PAPER 9 (ANSWER)

1----d

Right paratracheal stripe in chest x-ray is no more than 5 mm thick. There is no left paratracheal stripe because the outer margin of the left tracheal wall is virtually never outlined(the lung is separated from the trachea by the aorta and other vessels). **(G)**

2----a

Azygo-esophageal line is below azygos arch.Below the azygos arch, the right lower lobe makes contact with the right wall of the oesophagus and the azygos vein as it ascends next to the oesophagus. This portion of the lung is known as the azygo-oesophageal recess, and the interface is known as the azygo-oesophageal line. (G)

3----e

Untreated, at least one-third of patients of primary spontaneous pneumothorax has recurrence on the ipsilateral side. (G)

4---e

Cystic fibrosis,asthma, Chronic obstructive pulmonary disease, AIDS, Endometriosis (catamenial pneumothorax), Cavitary pneumonia, Tuberculosis, Pneumatocoele are other causes of spontaneous ,secondary pneumothorax in adult. **(G)**

5----b (Chapter 14,G)

6---d (Chapter 14, G)

7----a

Lymphadenopathy is the most common manifestation of primary tuberculosis in children and occurs with or without pneumonia. (Chapter 15, G)

8----c

Residual pleural change is unusual in pleural effusion of primary tuberculosis,.Pleural thickening and calcification is much more commonly due to a tuberculous empyema seen with post-primary disease. (Chapter 15,G)

9---e

At an early stage of the disease, HRCT can demonstrate airway abnormalities in patients who are asymptomatic and have normal pulmonary function and a normal chest radiograph. In patients with more advanced disease, HRCT is superior to chest radiography in detecting bronchiectasis and mucous plugging. (Chapter 16,G)

10---c

Most common acute changes of ABPA are transient consolidation, mucoid impaction and atelectasis. Atelectasis is subsegmental, segmental or lobar and has a tendency to recur in the same area. (Chapter 16,G)

11----e

The vertebral column appears progressively denser inferiorly in lower lobe collapse whereas normally the converse is true. (Chapter 17,G)

12---c

The 'superior triangle sign' refers to a triangular density to the right of the mediastinum seen in right lower lobe collapse due to displacement of anterior junctional structures.

The 'flat waist sign' is seen in extensive collapse of the left lower lobe and describes flattening of the contours of the aortic knuckle and main pulmonary artery due to cardiac rotation and displacement to the left.(Chapter 17, G)

13---e

T2 tumour -----Metastasis to ipsilateral mediastinal lymph nodes and subcarinal lymph nodes. (Chapter 18,G)

14---c (Chapter 18, G)

15----e (Chapter 18,G)

16----d

In general, NSIP may be distinguished from UIP on CT by a more prominent component of ground-glass attenuation and a finer reticular pattern in the absence of honeycombing. Fibrosis is usually of uniform temporality (in comparison to UIP). (Chapter 19, G)

17----c

Pleural plaques are not associated with significantly impaired lung function. Diffuse pleural thickening have a significant reduction in forced vital capacity (FVC) and gas transfer (DL_{co}). (Chapter 19, G)

18----b

On a chest radiograph the most frequent feature of COP is patchy, often subpleural and basal, areas of consolidation with preservation of lung volumes. The areas of airspace consolidation have a propensity to progress and change location over time. (Chapter 19,G)

19----d

Pleural effusions is not seen in ARDS. (CHAPTER 20 –G)

20----d (CHAPTER 20 ,G)

21---e (CHAPTER 6 ,G)

22---e

Cavitation is generally regarded as the classical radiological finding in pulmonary Wegener's granulomatosis and the demonstration of this sign is a useful pointer to the diagnosis .However, cavitation is by no means an invariable feature and thus, the absence of this sign should not preclude a diagnosis of Wegener's granulomatosis. (CHAPTER 21 ,G)

23----c

Consolidation in COP has a propensity for the sub-pleural and/or peribronchovascular regions in around two-thirds of patients. Cavitation is only rarely seen. Multifocal areas of ground-glass opacification with a surrounding rim of consolidation (known as the 'reverse halo' sign) is on CT scan. (CHAPTER 21,G)

24----a

The left atrium usually receives the four pulmonary veins at the 'corners' of its posterior surface. .(CHAPTER 22 ,G)

25----e

Anomalous pulmonary venous drainage causes large right atrium (CHAPTER 22,G)

26---c

The feature that best characterizes left ventricular morphology is fibrous continuity of the entry atrioventricular valve and the exit semilunar valve, due to the lack of any conus or infundibulum. (CHAPTER 22,G)

27----e

TOF shows oligaemia . (CHAPTER 23 ,G)

28----a (CHAPTER 23 ,G)

29---d

The Beall and Starr–Edwards 6500 series belong to Central caged disc occluder valve categories (CHAPTER 24,G)

30---e

Carpentier–Edwards ,the Hancock and the Ionescu–Shiley valves are bioprostheses. (CHAPTER 24,G)

31---e

MDCT can accurately determine CABG patency . (CHAPTER 25 .G)

32---a

There is high signal on T2-weighted image in recent myocardial infarction. Delayed contrast enhancement (DE-MRI) or high T2 signal is not specific to myocardial infarction and can be seen in other conditions causing myocardial damage, such as sarcoidosis or myocarditis. (CHAPTER 25,G)

33---e (CHAPTER 6 ,G)

34----e (CHAPTER 6 ,G)

35---e (CHAPTER 6,G)

36---a

Proposed upper limit of normal for mediastinal width is 8 cm and ratio of the mediastinal width to chest width at the level of the aortic arch is 0.25.(CHAPTER 27 ,G)

37----c (CHAPTER 27,G)

38----e (CHAPTER 28 ,G)

39----d

Retrieval of vena cava filter is via the jugular route, the right jugular vein being the ideal choice. (CHAPTER 28 ,G)

40----a (CHAPTER 64 ,G)

41----c (CHAPTER 64 ,G)

42-----a

Homogenous calcification ,ring calcification and popcorn calcification indicate of benign pathology.However lung metastases from osteogenic sarcoma are typically calcified in homogenous pattern.(Hagga)

43----e

The feeding vessel sign consists of a nodule or focal opacity that demonstrates a vessel leading to it .The presence of a feeding veseel indicates either that the lesion occurs in close proximity to small pulmonary vessels or the lesion has a hematogenous origin.(Hagga)

44---e

BOOP is predominantly lower lung disease (Webb)

45----d (Webb)

46----e

Myocardial iron overload cause diffuse reduction in contraction, decreased myocardial signal. (CHAPTER 22 ,G)

47---e

Thallioum 201 has long physical life . (CHAPTER 22 ,G)

48---b(CHAPTER 23 ,G)

49----e

Multilevel cine-MRA is probably the most accurate method for comprehensively assessing ventricular function. (CHAPTER 25,G)

50----b

The sinus venosus defect is found at the junction of either of the caval veins and the right atrium. The sinus venosus defect is often associated with partial anomalous pulmonary venous drainage. (CHAPTER 23 .G)

TEST PAPER 10

1.All are true regarding pulmonary artery except
a.The main PA measures upto 20mm in diameter in normal subjects
b.measurement made near the level of its bifurcation at right angles to the long axis of the PA
c.the PA is usually smaller than the adjacent aorta
d.the right and left pulmonary arteries size is approx. of equal size
e.the diameter of a small PA and its neighboring bronchus is of approx. equal size within the lung

2.A male patient of 55yrs was suffering from progressive shortness breath and a dry cough for more than 3-4 months.On examination finger clubbing and late inspiratory crackles is found .There is restrictive pattern of PFT and impaired gas exchange.All CT findings may be suggestive of idiopathic pulmonary fibrosis except
a. bibasilar reticulation
b.honecombing
c.central predominance of lesions
d.subpleural predominance of lesions
e.mediastinal lymphadenopathy

3.All are true regarding Bronchopulmonary sequestration (BPS) except
a. a mass of functioning lung tissue
b. does not communicate with the normal bronchial tree
c.receives its vascular supply from the systemic circulation
d. The in utero US appearance is of a solid, well-defined highly echo-reflective mass
e. The arterial supply is often difficult to visualize on colour flow Doppler

4.All are true regarding congenital lobar emphysema except
a. marked overaeration of a single pulmonary lobe
b. usually in the right middle lobe
c. compression of the remaining lobes of the lung
d. contralateral mediastinal shift
e. spontaneous resolution may occur

5.All are true regarding CT of aortic dissection except
a. intramural haematoma seen as areas of high attenuation
b. dissection flap visible as a linear track of high attenuation (from intimal calcification) within the aortic lumen on NECT
c. the dissection flap seen as a band of low attenuation on CECT

d. Injection of contrast medium via the left upper limb preferred

e. cobweb sign seen in false lumen

6.Features of false lumen that separate true lumen are all except

a. The false lumen usually tracks around the convexity of the aortic arch

b.false lumen is more often smaller than true lumens

c.The outer wall of the false lumen produces an acute angle at its junction with the dissection flap

d.linear strands of low attenuation within the false lumen (cobweb sign)

e. the true lumen shows continuity with the nondissected aorta.

7.All are true except

a. Persistent fetal circulation is seen in meconium aspiration syndrome

b. The most common cardiac cause of respiratory distress in neonate is a PDA

c. the left atrial-to-aortic root diameter ratio greater than 1.4 on day 3 in an otherwise normal heart is indicative of a haemodynamically significant PDA

d. Radiographic changes in survivors of uncomplicated RDS are very common

e.Approximately 80% of infants will have a PDA during the first 4 d of life

8.All are true regarding thymus except

a.thymus in newborn may cause abnormally wide or misshapen mediastinum

b. normal 'thymic rebound' may simulate mediastinal mass

c. The normal thymus displace the trachea posteriorly

d. The thymus is of lower attenuation than other mediastinal structures

e. The normal thymus has a uniform reflectivity on US

9.A dissection with thrombosed false lumen may be differentiated from an aneurysm with calcified mural thrombus by

a. High attenuation within the false lumen on unenhanced images

b. a dissection tends to spiral as it passes along the aorta whereas thrombus maintains a constant relationship with the aortic wall

c. Mural thrombus arising in an aneurysm tends to have an irregular internal border whilst a dissection has a smooth internal border

d. calcification of the intima may be identified at the periphery of the thrombus in an aneurysm

e.all

10.All are true regarding aortic dissection except

a. CECT allows the detection of the dissection flap in 99 of cases

b. High-speed pulse sequences are mandatory for vascular MRI imaging

c. TOE provide haemodynamic information about flow in the true and false lumen

d. Intravascular ultrasound has been useful in both the diagnosis and intervention of aortic dissection

e. transducer(12.5MHz) of intravascular ultrasound is used once

11.All are true regarding systemic supply to lungs except
a. severe right ventricular outlet obstruction
b. usually secondary to a severe TGA or pulmonary atresia
c. no main pulmonary artery is visible
d. the peripheral vascular pattern is often disorganized
e.may resemble interstitial lung disease

12.All are causes of uneven pulmonary vascularity except
a. bullae, emphysema
b. Macleod's syndrome,pulmonary arteriovenous fistulas.
c.previous pulmonary resection and pulmonary embolism.
d.Blalock–Taussig shunt and pulmonary artery stenosis
e.All

13.All are true regarding right coronary artery except
a. the right coronary artery (RCA) lie in the anterior atrioventricular groove
b. The RCA form the inverted U-loop of the crux
c. first branch is usually the conus branch
d.the second branch is the sinus node artery
e. the sinus node artery arises from the RCA in about one- third of cases

14.All are true regarding right coronary artery except

a. acute marginal branches supply the right ventricle.
b. the posterior descending coronary artery passes in the inferior interventricular groove on the inferior surface of the heart
c. the posterior descending coronary artery supply the lower part of the ventricular septum and the adjacent ventricular walls
d. The posterior descending branch can be recognized by inverted U-loop.
e. the atrioventricular nodal branch arise from RCA at the apex of the inverted 'U' of the crux .

15.The most common malignant tumour of the heart
a. Rhabdomyomas
b. Angiosarcoma
c.fibroma
d.lipoma
e.sarcomas

16. Aortic coarctation and/or pulmonary artery stenosis is noted in
a. Trisomy chromosome 21
b. Turner's syndrome
c. thalidomide syndrome
d. Holt–Oram syndrome
e. Ellis van Creveld syndrome

17.ASD is noted in
a. Trisomy chromosome 21
b. Turner's syndrome
c. thalidomide syndrome
d. Holt–Oram syndrome
e. Ellis van Creveld syndrome

18.Usually the most accurate method for imaging valve disease

a. transoesophageal echocardiography
b.subcostal echocardiography
c. supraternal echocardiography
d. apical echocardiography
e. right parasternal echocardiography

19.All are lung parenchymal changes in sarcoidosis except
a. parenchymal abnormalities and the nodal enlargement progresses in unison
b. rounded or irregular nodules 2–4 mm in diameter in 75–90%
c. patchy airspace consolidation in 10-20%
d. predominantly in the peribronchovascular regions of the middle and upper lungs zones
e. unusually coarse permanent fibrotic shadowing

20.All are HRCT finding of sarcoidosis except
a. peribronchovascular,subpleural distribution
b. perilymphatic distribution
c. small well-defined nodules (1-5mm)
d. fibrosis
e.a mid and lower zone distribution

21.All are true regarding parenchymal involvement of lung except
a. comparatively rare at initial presentation (10-15%)
b. three times more frequent in Hodgkin's lymphoma than in non-Hodgkin's lymphoma
c. The areas of pulmonary consolidation often radiate from the hila or mediastinum without conforming to segmental anatomy
d. non-Hodgkin's lymphoma of MALT type is the most frequently encountered form of primary lymphoma of lung
e. Pleural effusions are common in MALT lymphoma

22.All are true regarding pulmonary metastases except
a. one or more discrete pulmonary nodules usually in the inner portions of the lungs
b. The nodules usually spherical and well defined
c. usually from breast, gastrointestinal tract, kidney, testes, head and neck tumours
d. Cavitation occasionally seen
e. Calcification very unusual

23.All are true regarding emphysema except
a. Emphysema associated with α_1-antitrypsin deficiency is centrilobular in variety
b. The main radiographic manifestations are overinflation and alterations in the lung vessels
c. Signs of overinflation are the best predictors of the presence and severity of emphysema
d. Centrilobular emphysema is strongly associated with cigarette smoking.
e.In Panlobular emphysema Pathological changes are distributed throughout the lungs in Panlobular emphysema

24.All are signs of overinflation except

a. the height of the right lung being greater than 29.9 cm
b.location of the right hemidiaphragm at or below the anterior aspect of the seventh rib,
c.flattening of the hemidiaphragm,
d.norrowing of the retrosternal space,
e.widening of the sternodiaphragmatic angle and narrowing of the transverse cardiac diameter

25.All are true regarding tuberculosis except

a. Resolution of abnormal opacities suggest a satisfactory response to treatment
b.decrease in cavity size suggest a satisfactory response to treatment
c.volume loss from fibrosis is not the feature of satisfactory response to treatment
d. Extension of opacities on treatment raise the question of drug-resistant tuberculosis
e.incomplete resolution on treatment raise the question of drug-resistant tuberculosis

26.All are true regarding bronchogenic cyst except

a. usually solitary asymptomatic mediastinal masses
b. usually in contact of the carina or main bronchi,frequently project into the middle and/or posterior mediastinum
c. Most are unilocular and do not have a lobulated outline
d. Calcification of the wall or of the cyst contents is very common.

e. contents of uniform CT attenuation close to that of water (0 HU)

27.Lesions that push the carina forward and the oesophagus backward is /are

a. Foregut duplication cysts
b. thyroid masses
c.an aberrant left pulmonary artery
d.a+b
e.a+b+c

28.All are true regarding pleural thickening except

a. most commonly located in the non-dependent parts of the pleural cavity
b. On ultrasound, benign pleural thickening is not reliably detected unless it is 1 cm or more thick.
c. CT is very sensitive at detecting pleural thickening
d. benign pleural thickening is most easily assessed on the inside of the ribs on CT scan
e. fixed shadowing of water density

29.All are true regarding pleural plaques in asbestos exposure

a.often multifocal
b. undergo hyaline transformation,
c. may calcify/ ossify
d. most commonly found along the lower thorax and on the diaphragmatic pleura
e.diffuse pleural thickening is not seen

30.Modified Blalock–Taussig (BT) shunt for TOF refers to

a. the innominate artery and the left pulmonary artery
b. the innominate artery and the right pulmonary artery

c. the aorta and the right pulmonary artery

d. the aorta and the left pulmonary artery

e. the left pulmonary and the right pulmonary artery

31.All are features of active tuberculosis except

a.miliary disease

b.low density and rim enhancing hilar /mediastinal lymph nodes

c.pleural effusion

d.bronchopleural fistula and empyema necessitates

e.all

32.advantages of CT in tuberculosis is/are

a.in detection and characterization of subtle parenchymal and mediastinal disease

b.for distinguishing parenchymal cavities from areas of cystic bronchiectasis in association with lung fibrosis

c.detection of endobronchial spread of disease

d.reveal miliary disease when chest disease is normal

e.all

33.All are true regarding ILO classification for the pneumoconioses except

a. Irregular opacities are classified as s, t, or u

b. Rounded opacities are classified as p,q,r

c. Large opacities (> 10 mm) are graded as A, B and C

d. Profusion of the opacities is classified into four categories (0–3

e. the size of r opacity is (1.5-3 mm)

34.All are true regarding pulse sequences except

a. In spin-echo images the myocardium and vascular wall appear bright and the blood is dark

b. Gradient-echo imaging , blood produces a dark signal

c. Gradient-echo imaging allowing the acquisition of cine loops

d. Cine acquisitions are useful for the assessment of valves and regional contractile function of the myocardium

e. Phase-shift velocity mapping is based on phase component of the MR signal

35.Quantification of myocardial contraction can be done by

a. Myocardial tagging

b. MR velocity mapping.

c. Spin-echo imaging

d. Myocardial tagging and MR velocity mapping.

e. MR velocity mapping and Spin-echo imaging

36.Usually symptomatic vascular rings are all except

a. Double aortic arch

b. Right aortic arch with right descending aorta + aberrant left subclavian artery + persistent left arterial duct

c. Left aortic arch with right descending aorta + right arterial ductus

d. Left pulmonary sling

e. Left aortic arch + aberrant right subclavian artery

37.Williams' syndrome of infantile hypercalcaemia is associated with

a. congenital supravalvular aortic stenosis

b.congenital mitral stenosis

c. congenital tricuspid stenosis

d. congenital aortic regurgitation

e. congenital mitral regurgitation

38.All are true regarding cardiac tumours except

a. Metastatic tumours to the heart and pericardium are 2–4 times more common than primary heart tumours

b. Among primary cardiac tumours, benign tumours are more common than malignancy

c. CT allow tissue diagnosis of lipomas

d. transvenous spreadfrom the inferior vena cava to heart noted in renal or hepatic tumours

e. Myxomas are the most common cardiac primary tumour

39. CT features of a malignant nature of a cardiac neoplasm are

a. wide attachment to the wall of the heart

b.destruction of the cardiac chamber wall

c.limited to one cardiac chamber

d.invasion of the pericardium

e. extension into the pulmonary artery, pulmonary vein, or cava

40.All aretrue regarding angina pectoris except

a. Pain with spontaneous onset associated with ST segment elevation is termed Prinzmetal's or variant angina

b. Angina pectoris with apparently completely normal coronary arteries is known as syndrome X

c. perfusion defects noted on stress that fill in at rest in Thallium-201 scintigraphy

d. stress and rest images need to be acquired on different days in Thallium-201 scintigraphy

e. may occur in severe aortic stenosis and in hypertropic cardiomyopathy

41.All arer true regarding Dressler syndrome except

a. pleuritis (small pleural effusion)

b. pneumonitis (ill-defined basal lung shadows)

c. pericarditis

d. no role of aspirin

e. noted about 10–30 d after myocardial infarction or cardiac surgery

42.All are true regarding eventeration except

a. the normal diaphragmatic muscle replaced by a thin layer of connective tissue

b.broken continuity

c.marked left sided predominance in total eventeration

d. Partial eventration produce bulge in the dome

e. cause of respiratory distress in the newborn

43.All are true regarding diaphragm except

a. Unequal excursion of the two hemidiaphragms is less than 10 mm in most normal people

b. Bochdalek defects through the pleuroperitoneal canal occur along the anterior aspect of the diaphragm

c. Bochdalek the hernia are mostly occur on the left side

d. Morgagni hernia presents in adulthood as an anterior opacity at the right cardiophrenic angle

e. asymptomatic small Bochdalek hernias are present in 6% of otherwise normal adults

44.All are true regarding mediastinal lesions except

a. Oesophageal perforation is the most frequent cause of acute mediastinitis

b. Fibrosing mediastinitis is usually due to previous infection from histoplasmosis or tuberculosis

c.calcification is seen in fibrosing mediastinitis caused by lymphoma

d. haemorrhage produces an increase in the mediastinal diameter

e.dilatation of esophagus in fibrosing mediastnitis is noted

45.Continuous diaphragm sign is seen in

a. Mediastinal haemorrhage

b. Mediastinal emphysema

c. Fibrosing mediastinitis

d.diaphragmatic hernia

e.pericardial effusion

46.All are true regarding mediastinal lesions except

a. Oesophageal perforation is the most frequent cause of acute mediastinitis

b. Fibrosing mediastinitis is usually due to previous infection from histoplasmosis or tuberculosis

c.calcification is seen in fibrosing mediastinitis caused by lymphoma

d. haemorrhage produces an increase in the mediastinal diameter

e.dilatation of esophagus in fibrosing mediastnitis is noted

47.All are true regarding obliterative bronchiolitis except

a. mosaic perfusion on CT

b. vessels have the same calibre in both high and normal attenuation areas

c. Swyer–James or MacLeod syndrome, which is a variant form of postinfectious obliterative bronchiolitis affecting predominantly one lung.

d. CT technique for the assessment of air trapping is based on postexpiratory thin-section images

e. Objective measurement of air trapping can be done using CT densitometry.

48.Generally ,the smallest structures visible on HRCT range from

a.0.1-0.3mm

b.0.3-0.5mm

c.0.5-0.8mm

d.0.8-1.0mm

e.1.0-1.2mm

49.The presence of irregular interfaces between the aerated lung parenchyma and bronchi,vessels or plerural surfaces is reffered as

a.sagging sign

b.the interface sign

c.beaded sign

d.spiculated sign

e.romantic sign

50.All are true of peribronchovascular interstitial

thickening except
a.appear as increase in bronchial wall thickening on HRCT
b.appear as an increase in diameter of pulmonary artery branches on HRCT
c.equivalent to peribronchial cuffing in chest x ray
d.smooth variety typical of lymphatic spread of carcinoma
e.nodular variety seen in pulmonary edema

TEST PAPER 10 (ANSWER)

1---a
The main PA measures upto 30mm in diameter in normal subjects.(Webb)

2----c
In IPF ,lesions show peripheral and subpleural predominance .Evidence of fibrosis in form of traction bronchiectasis and bronchiolectasis ,intralobular interstitial thickening ,irregular interlobular septal thickening and honeycombing.(Webb)

3----a
Bronchopulmonary sequestration (BPS) represents a mass of nonfunctioning lung tissue. **(CHAPTER 64 ,G)**

4---b
 Congenital lobar emphysema is characterized by marked overaeration of a single pulmonary lobe, usually an upper lobe, less commonly the right middle lobe. **(CHAPTER 64,G)**

5----d
Injection of contrast medium via the left upper limb should be avoided as the very high attenuation from contrast medium within the left brachiocephalic vein can produce streak artefact across the aortic arch, potentially causing diagnostic difficulty . (CHAPTER 27,G)

6----b
The false lumen usually tracks around the convexity of the aortic arch and is more often than not the larger of the two lumens. Occasionally, linear strands of low attenuation may be seen within the false lumen (cobweb sign). These represent residual strands of media incompletely sheared away at the time of dissection. (CHAPTER 27 ,G)

7----d
Radiographic changes in survivors of uncomplicated RDS are uncommon and usually consist of mild linear shadowing representing fibrosis or deep pleural fissuring. **(CHAPTER 64 ,G)**

8----c
The normal thymus is said not to displace the trachea posteriorly unlike a true anterior mediastinal mass. **(CHAPTER 64 ,G)**

9---e (CHAPTER 27 ,G)

10---a
Contrast-enhanced CT allows the detection of the dissection flap in 70% of cases. (CHAPTER 27,G)

11---b
Systemic supply to the lungs develops in situations where there is severe right ventricular outlet obstruction (usually secondary to a severe Tetralogy of Fallot or pulmonary atresia). (CHAPTER 6,G)

12---e (CHAPTER 6 ,G)
13---e
The sinus node artery arises from the RCA in about two- third of cases. . (CHAPTER 25,G)
14---d
The posterior descending branch can be recognized by the straight, vertical septal vessels arising from it. (CHAPTER 25 ,G)
15----b (CHAPTER 24 ,G)
16---b (CHAPTER 23 ,G)
17---d (CHAPTER 23 ,G)
18----a (CHAPTER 22 ,G)
19---a
In sarcoidosis ,characteristically, parenchymal abnormalities appear as the nodal enlargement is subsiding (in lymphoma such abnormalities tend to progress in unison). (Chapter 19, G)
20---e
The combination of a peribronchovascular, subpleural distribution, small well-defined nodules, fibrosis and a mid and upper zone distribution are the features most helpful in making a diagnosis of sarcoidosis. (Chapter 19,G)
21----a
Parenchymal involvement is comparatively rare at initial presentation (10–15% of cases), but it becomes considerably more common as the disease progresses. Pleural effusions are common except in MALT lymphoma. (Chapter 18, G)

22-----a
In pulmonary metastases,one or more discrete pulmonary nodules are usually noted in in the outer portions of the lungs. (Chapter 18, G)
23---- a
Panlobular emphysema is the type of emphysema that occurs in α_1-antitrypsin deficiency and in familial cases. (Chapter 16, G)
24-----d
Widening of the retrosternal space is a sign of overinflation. (Chapter 16,G)
25----c
Volume loss from fibrosis suggest of satisfactory response to treatment. (Chapter 15,G)
26---d
Calcification of the wall or of the cyst contents is rare. Rarely, the cyst may show uniformly high density, probably due to a high protein content, or very high density indicating a very high calcium content (milk of calcium) within the fluid. (Chapter 14, G
27---e (Chapter 14,G)
28---a
Pleural thickening is most commonly located in the dependent parts of the pleural cavity . Viewed en profile, it appears as a band of soft tissue density up to approximately 10-mm thick, more or less parallel to the chest wall and with a sharp lung interface. En face, it causes ill-defined, veil-like shadowing. Blunting of the

costophrenic angle, often with tenting of the diaphragm, is a common finding. **(G)**

29---d
Diffuse pleural thickening is a manifestation of asbestos exposure. **(G)**

30---b (CHAPTER 23,G)

31------e (Webb)

32----e(Webb)

33----e
Rounded or nodular opacities are graded as p (< 1.5 mm diameter), q (1.5–3 mm), or r (3–10 mm). Irregular opacities are classified as s, t, or u, using the same size criteria. (Chapter 19, G)

34----b
Gradient-echo imaging blood produces a higher signal (white blood imaging). (CHAPTER 22,G)

35---d (CHAPTER 22 ,G)

36---e
Usually asymptomatic vascular rings are Left aortic arch + aberrant right subclavian artery, Left aortic arch with right descending aorta, Right aortic arch with right descending aorta + mirror image branching, Right aortic arch with right descending aorta + left aberrant subclavian artery, Right aortic arch with right descending aorta + isolation of left subclavian artery. (CHAPTER 23,G)

37----a (CHAPTER 23 ,G)

38---a
Metastatic tumours to the heart and pericardium are 20–40 times more common than primary heart tumours. (CHAPTER 24 ,G)

39---c
Involvement of more than one cardiac chamber is feature of malignant nature of cardiac neoplasm. (CHAPTER 24 ,G)

40----d
Stress and rest images need to be acquired on different days in SestaMIBI scintigraphy. SestaMIBI can be used in the acute phase of myocardial infarction to reveal perfusion deficits within the myocardium and their evolution over time, as well as in the assessment of angina. (CHAPTER 25 ,G)

41----d
Dressler s syndrome usually responds dramatically to aspirin or steroids, a useful distinguishing feature. (CHAPTER 25 ,G)

42----b
In eventration a part of the normal diaphragmatic muscle is replaced by a thin layer of connective tissue and a few scattered muscle fibres The unbroken continuity differentiates it from diaphragmatic hernia. **(G)**

43----b
Bochdalek defects through the pleuroperitoneal canal occur along the posterior aspect of the diaphragm. **(G)**

44----c
Calcification of hilar or mediastinal lymphnodes is noted in histoplasmosis/tuberculosis, which is an important feature for differentiating fibrosing mediastinitis from other infiltrative disorders of the mediastinum, such

as lymphoma and metastatic carcinoma. (Chapter 14,G)

45---b

In Mediastinal emphysema ,air may track extraserosally on either side of the diaphragm, which is occaisionally seen as a continuous line of transradiancy known as the 'continuous diaphragm sign'. (Chapter 14,G)

46-----c

Calcification of hilar or mediastinal lymphnodes is noted in histoplasmosis/tuberculosis, which is an important feature for differentiating fibrosing mediastinitis from other infiltrative disorders of the mediastinum, such as lymphoma and metastatic carcinoma. (Chapter 14, G)

47----b

The vessels within areas of decreased attenuation in obliterative bronchiolitis on thin-section CT may be of markedly reduced calibre, they are not distorted as in emphysema. The lung areas of decreased attenuation related to decreased perfusion can be patchy or widespread. They are poorly defined or sharply demarcated, giving a geographical outline, and represent a collection of affected secondary pulmonary lobules. Redistribution of blood flow to the normally ventilated areas causes increased attenuation of lung parenchyma in these areas. The patchwork of abnormal areas of low attenuation and normal lung or less diseased areas, appearing normal in attenuation or hyperattenuated, gives the appearance of mosaic attenuation. The vessels in the abnormal hypoattenuated areas are reduced in calibre, whereas the vessels in normal areas are increased in size; the resulting pattern is called mosaic perfusion. The difference in vessel size between low and high attenuation areas allows the mosaic perfusion pattern to be distinguished from mosaic attenuation due to an infiltrative lung disease with patchy distribution, in which the vessels have the same calibre in both high and normal attenuation areas. (Chapter 16, G)

48----b (Webb)

49-----b (Webb)

50----e

Pulmonary edema give rise to smooth peribronchovascular interstitial thickening.(Webb)

TEST PAPER 11

1.All are true regarding fibrothorax /diffuse pleural thickening

a. a smooth uninterrupted pleural density that extends over at least one-quarter of the chest wall

b. extends more than 8 cm in the craniocaudal direction, 5 cm laterally and a thickness of more than 3 mm on CT scan

c. Extensive calcification favours previous tuberculosis or empyema

d. Asbestos exposure-related fibrothorax is usually bilateral and heavily calcified

e. mesothelioma, lymphoma and leukaemia may cause fibrothorax

2. The useful features that indicate malignant as opposed to benign pleural thickening are all except

a. circumferential thickening

b. nodularity

c. parietal thickening of more than 1 cm,

d. involvement of the mediastinal pleura

e. Signal hypointensity with long TR sequences

3.All are true regarding mediastinal cysts except

a. The mediastinal pancreatic pseudocyst is almost always in the anterior mediastinum adjacent to the oesophagus

b. Oesophageal duplication cysts has thicker wall and more tubular appearance than bronchogenic cyst

c. Neurenteric cysts are typically associated with vertebral body anomalies such as butterfly or hemivertebra.

d. neurenteric cyst is located in the posterior mediastinum between the oesophagus and the spine

e. Oesophageal duplication cysts usually present first in childhood

4.The best investigation for neurogenic tumours is

a.CECT

b.USG

c.Nuclear scan

d.MRI

e.PET scan

5.Central target calcification with surrounding soft tissue opacity (Target lesions) in chest X-ray is suggestive of

a. Cryptococcosis (torulosis)

b. Histoplasmosis

c. Coccidioidomycosis

d. Aspergillus infection

e. Protozoal infections

6.All are radiological appearance of hydatid disease of lung except

a. the air crescent

b. an air–fluid level

c. water lily sign

d. camalote sign

e.corona sign

7.Alterations in lung vessels noted in emphysema are all except

a. arterial depletion

b. vessels of normal(occasionally increased) calibre in unaffected areas of the lung

c.absence or displacement of vessels caused by bullae

d.narrowing of branching angles of vessel

e.loss of side branches and vascular redistribution.

8.All are true regarding vanishing lung syndrome except

a. mainly seen in old men

b. the presence of large progressive upper lobe bullae

c. occupy a significant volume of a hemithorax

d. are often asymmetrical

e. also known as giant bullous emphysema/primary bullous disease of the lung

9.All are true regarding pulmonary metastases except

a. irregular edges of nodule are seen in with metastases from adenocarcinomas

b. Cavitation is a particular feature of metastases from squamous cell carcinoma

c. Calcification is seen in metastases from osteosarcoma and chondrosarcoma

d. metasetases from some choriocarcinomas and osteosarcomas may double its the volume in less than 30 d

e. visible calcification in the

pulmonary metastases from breast and colon is common

10.All are true regarding pulmonary metastases except

a.low KV techniques of chest x ray are routinely used

b.proper chest x ray detect most lung metastases above 1 cm in diameter

c. lesions 3-10mm in diameter is regularly demonstrated on CT

d. the probability of multiple noncalcified nodules being metastases on plain chest x ray is well over 90%

e. the probability of a pulmonary nodule seen solely on CT being a metastasis is as low as 50%.

11.All are true regarding hypersensitivity pneumonitis except

a. the fluctuating nature of changes on serial radiographs in acute stage

b. poorly defined, < 5 mm in diameter], centrilobular nodules ,seen throughout the lung

c. Ground-glass opacity is in the acute phase only

d. mosaic attenuation pattern

e. fibrosis with upper lobe retraction, reticular opacity, volume loss and honeycombing in chronic stage

12.All are true regarding Langerhans cell histiocytosis (LCH)

a. widespread, bilateral and usually symmetrical involvement of lung

b. nodules (few millimetres to 2 cm)

c. sparing of the extreme lung bases and anterior tips of the right middle lobe and lingula

d. pneumothorax

e.thin-walled cyst with oval shapes

13.Stress echocardiography uses

a.dopamine

b.dobutamine

c.nifedipine

d.propranolol

e.aminophylline

14.EBCT uses

a. an electronically steered beam of protons

b. an electronically steered beam of electrons

c. an electronically steered beam of neutrons

d. an electronically steered beam of positrons

e. an electronically steered beam of neutrinos

15.A common atrial chamber is noted in

a. Trisomy chromosome 21

b. Turner's syndrome

c. thalidomide syndrome

d. Holt–Oram syndrome

e. Ellis van Creveld syndrome

16. The first-line investigation of congenital heart disease is

a.chest xray

b.echocardiography

c.MRI

d.PET

e.CT

17.The best imaging method to categorize various forms of cardiomyopathies

a.Echo

b .contrast enhanced CMR

c.MDCT

d.PET

e.Chest x ray

18.All are true of Hypertrophic cardiomyopathy (HCM) except

a. often familial

b. excessive hypertrophy of the right and left ventricular myocardium in all cases

c. upper interventricular septum is most affected in idiopathic hypertrophic subaortic stenosis

d. systolic anterior motion of the mitral valve (SAM).

e. similar pathological changes seen in Noonan's syndrome and Friedreich's ataxia

19.All are true regarding right coronary artery except

a. the right coronary artery (RCA) lie in the anterior atrioventricular groove

b. The RCA form the inverted U-loop of the crux

c. first branch is usually the conus branch

d.the second branch is the sinus node artery

e. the sinus node artery arises from the RCA in about one- third of cases

20.All are true regarding right coronary artery except

a. acute marginal branches supply the right ventricle.

b. the posterior descending coronary artery passes in the inferior interventricular groove on the inferior surface of the heart

c. the posterior descending coronary artery supply the lower part of the ventricular septum and the adjacent ventricular walls

d. The posterior descending branch can be recognized by inverted U-loop.

e. the atrioventricular nodal branch arise from RCA at the apex of the inverted 'U' of the crux .

21 The 'gold standard' for pre-therapeutic pulmonary arteriovenous malformation investigation is

a. CT (3D reconstructions)

b.MR Angiography

c.selective angiography

d.chest ray

e.PET

22.All are true regarding congenital pulmonary artery absence except

a. failure of development of the right or left sixth branchial arterial arch

b. short segment atresia of the proximal left or right pulmonary artery

c. distal segments of pulmonary artery are usually present

d. a small volume ipsilateral lung with air trapping

e. small ipsilateral hilum

23.All are true regarding management of aortic dissection except

a. Emergent surgical repair is indicated in all patients with Type A dissection

b. late surgery is recommended for patients with Marfan's syndrome with type B dissection

c. patients with type B dissection having persistent pain and/or progression are referred for either surgical or endovascular intervention

d. . Endovascular techniques has less morbidity and mortality in comparison to surgery

e. Acute type B dissections are the most appropriate group to treat by Placement of a stent graft

24.All are true regarding management of type B dissection

a. Contained rupture and Branch vessel ischaemia are the indications for stent or stent graft placement

b. stent graft placement may become the treatment of choice

c. Surgery is associated with mortality in excess of 50% in cases with end-organ ischaemia

d. In uncomplicated type B dissection surgery is initial treatment

e. Early surgery is recommended for patients with Marfan's syndrome

25.All are true except

a. At least five anterior rib ends should be visualized above the diaphragm before a chest radiograph can be considered adequate

b. Chest radiographs help detect the complications of bronchiolitis

c. Round pneumonia resolves very slowly with treatment

d. A poorly defined cardiac outline due to sublobar consolidation is often seen with *Bordetella pertussis*

e. Following clinical resolution of *Staphylococcus aureus* thin-walled 'ghost cavities' may persist for months

26.All are true except

a. The chest radiograph in tuberculous meningitis (TBM) is often normal

b. The right middle lobe may be due to tuberculosis

c. the lower lobes is more commonly affected lobe in infants with aspiration pneumonia

d.most common cause of pleural effusions in children is infection

e. the most common cause of the unilaterally opaque chest radiograph in children is infection

27..A 50 yrs old patient of mitral stenosis started discomfort and breathlessness for which he was admitted .The chesxt x ray shows cardiomegaly with hilar prominence .Pulmoray edema of cardiogenic natur was suspected .What may be other additional finding

a.patchy ground glass opacity

b.peribronchial cuffing

c.smooth subpleural /fissural thickening

d.smooth interlobular septal thickening

e.peripheral /upper lung predominance

28.A 26 yrs old patient is suffering from nonproductive cough ,fever and mild dyspnoe on exertion

.The chest x ray of patient showed a bilateral patchy ,diffuse airspace opacity ,most severe in the lung bases .BAL shows PAS + material .The finding which favour alveolar proteinosis is

a.crazy-paving appearance

b.honeycombing

c.hilar lymphadenopathy

d.pleural effusion

e.cardiomegaly

29.A patient experienced asbestos exposure for more than 10 yrs and is now revealing restrictive pattern on PFT.The patient is advised HRCT to detect the feature of asbestosis.The earliest abnormal findings recognizable on HRCT of this patient is

a.thickening of interlobular septa

b.intralobular interstitial thickening

c.subpleural dotlike opacities

d.traction bronchiectasis

e.honeycombing

30.The pattern of TB in HIV-positive patients differs from that in non-AIDS patients.findings more commonly seen in TB patients with the HIV-postivity is /are

a.diffuse disease

b.atypical infiltrates

c.mediastinal lymphadenopathy

d.miliary disease

e. cavitation

31.CT findings of TB found to be less common in HIV-positive patients include all except

a.cavitation and nodules 10-30 mm in diameter

b.findings of endobronchial spread of infection

c.diffuse

d.bronchial wall thickening

e.findings typical of postprimary infection

32.Halo sign (halo surrounding the nodule is of lower attenuation than the nodule itself) is noted in

a.tuberculoma

b.alveolar proteinosis

c.angioinvasive aspergillosis

d.pneumoconiosis

e.hypersencitivity pneumonitis

33.HIV –infected patients showing demonstration of PCP organisms in sputum undergoes HRCT. Findings suggestive of PCP is/are all except

a.patchy or diffuse ground glass opacity

b.central,perihilar or upper lobe predominance

c.massivew hilar adenopathy

d.thick-walled irregular septated cavities

e.thin-walled cysts

34.The Norwood procedure is surgical treatment of

a.TOF

b.Single ventricle

c. Hypoplastic left heart syndrome

d. double outlet right ventricle

e. Transposition of the great arteries

35.All are true except

a. Type III of TAPVD is most common type

b. pulmonary congestion is noted in type 111 TAPVD

c. atrialization of the proximal right ventricle is noted in Ebstein's anomaly

d. perforated fibromuscular septum is noted in cor triatrium

e. gross right atrial enlargement is noted in Ebstein's anomaly

36. The most frequent causes of sudden cardiac death in competitive young athletes.

a. hypertropic cardiomyopathy

b.arrhythmogenic right ventricular dysplasia

c.anomalous origin of the left coronary artery

d. hypertropic cardiomyopathy + arrhythmogenic right ventricular dysplasia

e. hypertropic cardiomyopathy + arrhythmogenic right ventricular dysplasia+ anomalous origin of the left coronary artery.

37.All are true regarding cardiovascular MRI except

a. Phase-contrast imaging is used for anatomical imaging

b. two forms of cardiac gating---- Prospective gating retrospective gating

c. Navigator techniques monitor respiratory motion

d. dobutamine or adenosine can be used for assessing myocardial ischaemia

e. Prospective gating detects the QRS complex of the ECG

38.The main indications for the use of contrast agents in CMR are
a. assessment of myocardial perfusion
b. contrast-enhanced MRA
c improved demarcation of normal and infarcted myocardium
d. delineation of viability after coronary occlusion
e.all

39.Right and left atrial isomerism is associated with all except
a. an endocardial cushion defect
b. atrioventricular septal defect (AVSD).
c. Bilateral superior vena cavae
d. Pulmonary stenosis/atresia
e. Anomalous pulmonary veins

40.All are true regarding Aortic coarctation except
a. narrowing in the thoracic aorta in the region of insertion of the arterial duct (aortic isthmus)
b. No risk of systemic hypertension even after surgical repair
c. Reassessment of collateral flow following treatment can be used to assess the success of the treatment
d. Three-dimensional contrast-enhanced MRA may display the severity and extent of involvement
e. Coarctation occurs in 6–8% of live CHD births

41.All are true except
a. deposition of elastic tissue on the inside of the left ventricle in Endocardial fibroelastosis
b. thickened endocardium appearing as white line on Echo in endocardial fibroelastosis
c. the left ventricle wall markedly thickened and irregular in outline on its inner aspect in Pompe disease
d. gross myocardial wall thinning in Fabry disease
e. doxorubicin the most likely cytotoxic drug to precipitate a syndrome of congestive cardiomyopathy

42. The imaging technique of choice for the diagnosis of intracardiac tumours
a.Echo
b .contrast enhanced CMR
c.MDCT
d.PET
e.Chest x ray

43.All are true regarding myocardial stunning except
a. abnormal ventricular function
b. the myocardium is viable
c.no recovery of left ventricular function during extended pharmacological stress testing
d. has contractile reserve
e. can regain normal function with revascularization

44.All are true regarding myocardial hibernation except
a. result from months or years of ischaemia
b.ventricular dysfunction revesible with revascularization
c. the affected myocardium shows contractile reserve
d. DE-MRI can be used to differentiate hibernating myocardium from infarct
e. Radionuclides is of no use in its study

45.All are used in ventilation scintigraphy of lunf except

144

a. ^{99m}Tc micro-aggregate albumin (MAA

b. krypton-81m

c. xenon-133

d. ^{99m}Tc-diethylenetriamine penta-acetic acid (DTPA)

e. 'technegas'

46.All are true regarding ventilation scintigraphy of lung except

a. ^{81m}Kr has a long half-life

b. emits high energy photons 190keV

c. can be continuously administered to the patient

d. the optimal imaging agent

e. expensive.

47.All are true of Alagille syndrome except

a. cause cholestasis

b. mutations in the JAG1 gene

c. Mid aortic coarctation

d. ocular defects

e. adult presentation

48.All are true regarding aortic occlusive disease except

a. Atherosclerosis is the predominant cause

b. affects a younger population than that of lower limb arterial disease

c. The infra-inguinal arteries characteristically involved

d. typically female,

e. a small infrarenal aorta and hypoplastic iliofemoral arteries

49. ^{99m}Tc-Pertechnetate study is done in

a. duplication cyst of the oesophagus

b. Bronchopulmonary sequestration

c. diaphragmatic hernia

d. aortic ring anomalies

e. Pericardial cysts

50.All are true regarding mediastinal mass except

a. m/c anterior mediastinal masses ---- nodal (lymphoma or leukaemia)

b. compression of the trachea noted with an anterior mass

c. Calcification in a middle or anterior mediastinal mass suggests a teratoma or hamartoma

d. a cystic mass in the middle mediastinum is most commonly a pericardial cyst

e. Calcification in a posterior mass suggests a sympathetic chain tumour

TEST PAPER 11(ANSWER)

1----d
Asbestos exposure-related fibrothorax is less common than pleural plaques and is usually the sequel of a benign exudative effusion. Asbestos exposure-related fibrothorax is usually bilateral and rarely calcified. (The Normal Chest Adam: Grainger & Allison's Diagnostic Radiology, 5th ed).

2----e
Signal hypointensity with long TR sequences is a reliable predictive sign of benign pleural disease. (G)

3----a
The mediastinal component of the pseudocyst is almost always in the posterior mediastinum adjacent to the oesophagus, having gained access to the chest via the oesophageal or aortic hiatus. CT is the optimal method of demonstrating these thin-walled cysts, which show continuity with the pancreas and any peripancreatic fluid collections. (Chapter 14, G)

4----d
The best investigation for neurogenic tumours is MRI. (Chapter 14,G)

5--- b
Central target calcification with surrounding soft tissue opacity (Target lesions) in chest X-ray is suggestive of Histoplasmosis.

(Chapter 15,G)

6----e (Chapter 15,G)

7----d
Alterations in lung vessels in emphysema include arterial depletion, whereas vessels of normal, or occasionally increased, calibre are present in unaffected areas of the lung, absence or displacement of vessels caused by bullae, widened branching angles with loss of side branches and vascular redistribution. (Chapter 16,G)

8---- a
Vanishing lung syndrome is mainly seen in young men. (Chapter 16,G)

9----e
Visible calcification in the pulmonary metastases from breast and colon is rare (Chapter 18,G)

10---a
The simplest technique for diagnosing pulmonary metastases is the plain postero-anterior (PA) and lateral chest radiograph. High-kV techniques are often used routinely, since substantial portions of the lungs are obscured on low-kV radiographs by overlying structures such as the diaphragm, heart, mediastinum, hila and ribs. (Chapter 18,G)

11----c

Ground-glass opacity is most common in the acute phase but may also be a feature of subacute and chronic hypersensitivity pneumonitis, especially if there is ongoing exposure. (Chapter 19,G)

12----e
The classical appearances of LCH on HRCT are nodules (ranging in size from a few millimetres to 2 cm), several of which show cavitation and have bizarre shapes. The typical nodules of LCH tend to show a predictable progression through the following stages: cavitation of the nodules, thin-walled cystic lesions, and finally emphysematous and fibrobullous destruction. (Chapter 19,G)

13---b (CHAPTER 22 ,G)

14---b
EBCT uses an electronically steered beam of electrons aimed at a series of tungsten rings to generate X-rays. (CHAPTER 22 ,G)

15----e (CHAPTER 23 ,G)

16---b (CHAPTER 23 ,G)

17----b (CHAPTER 24 ,G)

18----b
HCM is characterized by excessive hypertrophy of the left ventricular myocardium,right ventricle may be involved but not in all cases. (CHAPTER 24 ,g)

19----e
The sinus node artery arises from the RCA in about two- third of cases. . (CHAPTER 25 ,G)

20---d

The posterior descending branch can be recognized by the straight, vertical septal vessels arising from it. (CHAPTER 25,G)

21---c (CHAPTER 6 ,G)

22----d
The principal radiological features are a small volume ipsilateral lung without air trapping (air trpping in Macleod's syndrome). (CHAPTER 6 ,G)

23---b
Early surgery is recommended for patients with Marfan's syndrome with type B dissection. (CHAPTER 27 ,G)

24----d
In uncomplicated type B dissection (no evidence of rupture or branch vessel ischaemia) medical treatment is initially implemented, as both medical and emergent surgical management are associated with similar mortality rates. Patients who fail medical management (persistent pain and/or progression of dissection) or develop complications are referred for either surgical or endovascular intervention. Early surgery is recommended for patients with Marfan's syndrome. (CHAPTER 27 .G)

25----c
Round pneumonia resolves rapidly with treatment. The chest radiograph shows a rounded or spherical opacity with poorly defined margins, simulating a pulmonary mass. (CHAPTER 64.G)

26----c

The upper lobes is more commonly affected in infants with aspiration pneumonia . **(CHAPTER 64,G)**

27----e

Lesions of cardiogenic pulmonary edema shows predominance in dependent ,perihilar (Bat –wing)or lower lung predominance.(Webb)

28-----a (Webb)

29----c

The arliest abnormal findings recognizable on HRCT reflect the presence of centrilobular ,peribronchiolar fibrosis (dot like opacities ,subpleural curvilinear opacities.(Webb)

30----e (Webb)

31----c (Webb)

32----c (Webb)

33-----c (Webb)

34-----c (CHAPTER 23,G)

35----a

The infracardiac type (type111) is the least common variant and makes up approximately 12% of TAPVD cases.In total anomalous pulmonary venous drainage (TAPVD) the pulmonary veins coalesce posterior to the left atrium, but do not drain into it. Drainage from this venous confluence to the right atrium may be: (a) via either an ascending vein to the innominate vein, and then to the SVC (supracardiac, Type I) (b) the coronary sinus directly into the right atrium (cardiac, Type II); or (c) via a descending vein, which passes through the diaphragm into either the IVC or portal venous system (infracardiac, Type III) . (CHAPTER 23 ,G)

36----e

Hypertropic cardiomyopathy ,arrhythmogenic right ventricular dysplasia and anomalous origin of the left coronary artery are the most frequent causes of sudden cardiac death in competitive young athletes. (CHAPTER 23,G)

37-----a

Phase-contrast imaging is used to measure blood flow velocity. (CHAPTER 22,G)

38---e (CHAPTER 22 ,G)

39----e

Anomalous pulmonary veins, Double outflow right ventricle are not associated with left isomerism. Both right- and left-sided isomerism are associated with gut malrotation. (CHAPTER 23,G)

40----b

There is a risk of systemic hypertension, atherosclerosis and end-organ damage, even in patients who have undergone surgical repair. (CHAPTER 23,G)

41---d

Fabry's disease cause gross the myocardial wall thickening .(CHAPTER 24,G)

42---a (CHAPTER 24 ,G)

43----c (CHAPTER 25 ,G)

44----e (CHAPTER 25,G)

45---a

Perfusion (Q) scintigraphy (to assess the distribution of pulmonary blood flow) is performed using injection of microparticles (10–100μm) of

^{99m}Tc micro-aggregate albumin (MAA)(G)

46---a

^{81m}Kr has a short half-life and is expensive. It is the optimal imaging agent for this purpose as it emits high energy photons (190keV) and owing to its short half-life can be continuously administered to the patient, including during perfusion imaging. (CHAPTER 6,G)

47----e

Alagille syndrome often presents with clinical symptoms involving the liver during infancy and early childhood. Alagille syndrome is the most common form of the inherited disorders that cause cholestasis. Patients have distinctive facial features with deep set eyes, frontal bossing, bulbous tip of the nose, a down-turned mouth and a small mandible with pointed chin. (CHAPTER 27 ,G)

48---c

The infra-inguinal arteries are 'protected' by the aortic lesion and are characteristically disease free aortic occlusive disease. (CHAPTER 27 ,G)

49---a (CHAPTER 64 ,G)

50---d

A cystic mass in the middle mediastinum is most commonly a bronchogenic cyst. Foregut remnants (bronchogenic cysts, oesophageal duplication, neurenteric cyst) are due to failure of normal embryology as the primitive notocord, oesophagus, and trachea develop and separate.(CHAPTER 64 ,G)

TEST PAPER 12

1.All are true regarding pleural calcification except
a. calcification is irregular in tuberculous empyema and haemothorax
b. calcification in empyema is most common in the lower anterior half of the chest
c. calcification in empyema is usually unilateral
d. calcification in asbestosis occurs as more discrete collections within plaques
e. calcification in asbestosis is usually bilateral.

2.All are true regarding localized mesothelioma except
a.middle age
b.hypertrophic osteoarthropathy in more than 50% cases
c.two thirds benign in nature
d. positional variation with changes in posture and respiration
e.highly calcified

3.The most common tumours to arise in the posterior mediastinum
a. Neurenteric cysts
b. Oesophageal duplication cysts
c. Neurogenic tumours
d. Bronchogenic cysts
e.maignant lymphoma

4.All are true regarding peripheral nerve tumours in mediastinum except

a. typically originate in an intercostal nerve in the paravertebral region
b. bone changes in adjacent ribs ,vertebra,(such as thickened scalloped cortex) are diagnostic of a neurogenic lesion
c. The rib spaces and the intervertebral foramina may be widened by the tumour
d. target sign on T2-weighted images and shows uniform enhancement on MRI
e. foci of calcification never seen

5.All are radiological appearance of hydatid disease of lung except
a. rising sun sign
b. serpent sign
c. empty cyst sign
d. air bubble sign
e.Reigler s notch

6. All are radiological appearance of hydatid disease of lung except
a. a floating membrane (water lily sign, camalote sign)
b. an essentially dry cyst with crumpled membranes lying at its bottom (rising sun sign, serpent sign
c. a cyst with all its contents expectorated (empty cyst sign)
d. a double wall
e. Reigler s notch

7.The most accurate means of detecting emphysema and

150

determining its type and extent in vivo

a.x ray

b.HRCT

c.MRI

d.USG

e.nuclear scan

8. The most cost-effective and widely used method of screening for pulmonary metastases is

a.plain chest x ray

b.CT scan

c.PET

d.MRI

e.USG

9.All are true regarding lymphangitic carcinomatosis

a. fine reticulonodular shadowing

b. subpleural oedema

c. Pleural effusion rare

d. nonuniform, often nodular, thickening of the interlobular septa

e. bilateral symmetric pulmonary abnormality in blood borne cases

10.Endobronchial submucosal metastases are most commonly noted in primar tumour of all except

a.Melanoma

b.renal carcinoma

c.colorectal carcinoma

d.breast carcinoma

e.prostatic carcinoma

11.All are true regarding Lymphangioleiomyomatosis (LAM) except

a. almost exclusively in men

b. generalized, symmetrical,

reticular, or reticulonodular opacities

c. pneumothoraces in approximately 50%

d. Pleural effusions occur in 10–40% of patients

e. numerous thin-walled cysts

12.Deveplopment in MDCT favouring interest of cardiac CT is/are

a. fast tube rotation

b.ECG triggering of image acquisition

c.ECG controlled modulation of tube current

d.sophisticated post-processing

e.all

13.Cardiac abnormalities detected by CT without use of contrast is/are

a. lipomatous hypertrophy of the atrial septum

b.fatty degeneration of the myocardium

c. calcification (coronary artery, aneurysm, valves)

d. The position of implants

e. all

14.For accurate anatomical imaging of heart ,which sequence is used

a. Black blood' spin-echo images,

b. 'White blood' gradient-echo

c. Phase-contrast imaging

d. Contrast-enhanced MR angiography (MRA)

e. steady-state free precession (SSFP)

15. For cine imaging and quantification of ventricular

volumes, mass and function,which sequence is used

a. Black blood' spin-echo images,

b. 'White blood' gradient-echo

c. Phase-contrast imaging

d. Contrast-enhanced MR angiography (MRA)

e. steady-state free precession (SSFP)

16.The best technique to follow the natural history of the HCM

a. Serial measurement of left ventricle mass by MDCT

b. Serial measurement of left ventricle mass by CMR

c. Serial measurement of left ventricle mass by ECHO

d. Serial measurement of left ventricle mass by PET

e. Serial measurement of left ventricle mass by CHEST XRAY

17.The shape of left ventricle on ventriculography in HCM is

a.orange shaped

b.pear shaped

c.banana –shaped

d.lemon –shaped

e.apple shaped

18.All are true regarding coronary artery except

a. Dominance indicates the coronary artery that supplies the posterior descending branch to the inferior surface of the heart

b. left dominance noted in 85%

c. variations of dominance represents about 60% of all major congenital anomalies

d. Cx may originate from the RCA or as a separate artery from the right coronary sinus

e. Major congenital variants of coronary anatomy occur in about 1–2% of patients

19.All are true regarding coronary artery stenosis except

a. The normal coronary artery is a smooth, gently tapering, branching structure

b. Calcification indicates the presence of atherosclerosis

c. the greater the calcification the greater the likelihood of there being a stenosis in artery

d. A reduction of lumen diameter of over 50–60% is thought to represent a haemodynamically significant stenosis

e. arteriography tends to overrestimate the degree of atheroma and the severity of the stenosis.

20.All are associated with pulmonary artery stenosis except

a. rubella syndrome

b.William's syndrome

c.Ehlers–Danlos syndrome

d. no cardiac lesions

e. sausage-shaped arteries

21.All are causes of pulmonary artery mycotic aneurysm except

a. Infected ventricular shunts

b. Valvular bacterial endocarditis of right ventricle

c. Tuberculosis (Rasmussen aneurysm

d. Behçet's disease

e.all

22.All causes of acquired inflammatory aortitis except

a. giant cell arteritis

b.Buerger's, Behĉet's

c.Cogan's disease

d.Kawasaki diseases.

e. neurofibromatosis

23.All are true regarding Granulomatous vasculitis (Takayasu's disease) except

a. involves the aorta, its branches and the pulmonary arteries
b. varying degree of stenosis, occlusion, or dilatation of the involved vessels
c.more common in developed country including Japan
d. more in female
e. a disease of young adults

24.Mediastinal shift towards the abnormal side is noted in all except

a. Pulmonary agenesis or hypoplasia
b. Cystic congenital adenomatoid malformation
c. Scimitar syndrome (hypogenetic lung)
d. Bronchopulmonary sequestration (basal)
e. Swyer James (MacLeod) syndrome

25.The most common site of lodgement of foreign body is

a. the right bronchus intermedius
b.the right lower medial bronchus
c. the right lower lateral bronchus
d. the right lower basal bronchus
e. the right lower superior bronchus

26.A patient experienced asbestos exposure for more than 10 yrs and is now revealing restrictive pattern on PFT.The patient is advised HRCT to detect the feature of asbestosis.All are common features of asbestosis except

a.bilateral and often symmetrical changes
b.earliest change basal and posterior
c.subpleural lines and dots
d.ground glass opacity
e.parietal pleura thickening

27. A patient of 45yrs were exposed to prolonged asbestosis and developed rounded peripheral opacity abutting the pleural surface and shows dense enhancement with curving of pulmonary vessels into the edge of the lesion.The most likely diagnosis is

a.pulmonary carcinoma
b.mesothelioma
c.rounded atelectasis
d.hamatoma
e.carcinoid

28.All are true of ground glass opacity except

a.hazy increase in lung attenuation
b.does not obscure underlying vessel
c.due to morphological abnormality well resolved by HRCT
d.seen in PCP
e.seen in alveolar proteinosis

29. Ideal for imaging the RVOT and branch pulmonary arteries in post operative case of TGA

a. PET
b.chest x ray
c.MDCT

d. trans-thoracic echocardiography
e.MRI

30. All are true regarding congenitally corrected transposition of arteries except
a. atrioventricular discordance
b.no associated cardiac lesions
c. ventricle–arterial discordance
d. physiologically normal in terms of the pulmonary and systemic circuits
e. does not usually cause cyanosis

31. All are true except
a. In double outlet right ventricle, both great vessels emerge from the right ventricle
b. double outlet right ventricle part of 'Taussig–Bing' anomaly
c. the Rastelli procedure useful in the single ventricle
d. single arterial trunk arises from both ventricles in truncus arteriosus
e. In Type I, a short main pulmonary artery arises from the common trunk and subsequently divides

32. All are correctly matched operations except
a.TOF--- modified Blalock–Taussig (BT) shunt
b.Single ventricle ---Fontan operation
c.Single ventricle ---Glenn operation
d. double outlet right ventricle --- hemi-Fontan operation
e. Transposition of the great arteries---the Senning and Mustard procedure

33. All are causes of bilateral symmetrical elevation of diaphragm except
a. Diffuse pulmonary fibrosis

b. Lymphangitis carcinomatosa
c. Disseminated lupus erythematosus
d. Bilateral basal pulmonary emboli
e. Bilateral subpulmonary effusion

34. All are causes of unilateral elevation of dome of diaphragm except
a. Pulmonary hypoplasia
b. Pulmonary collapse
c.Disseminated lupus erythematosus
d. Phrenic nerve palsy
e. Eventration

35. Splitting of the trachea from the oesophagus is a characteristic of all except
a. thyroid masses
b.bronchogenic cysts
c.neurogenic tumours
d.oesophageal tumours
e. an aberrant origin of the left pulmonary artery

36. All are paravertebral masses except
a. Neurogenic lesions
b. neoplastic lymphadenopathy
c. extramedullary haematopoiesis
d. pancreatic pseudocyst
e. Aneurysms of the ascending aorta

37. All are true regarding mycobacterial tuberculosis in AIDS patients with advanced immunosuppression except
a. diffuse bilateral coarse reticulonodular opacities
b. Hilar and/or mediastinal adenopathy
c. a mid or lower lobe predominance of lesions
d.marked Cavitation

e. increasing mediastinal adenopathy and worsening or new lung opacities on use of HAART

38.All are true regarding pulmonary infections in AIDS patients

a. The principal chest radiographic abnormality of suspected cytomegalovirus pneumonia is a bilateral fine reticular pattern

b. coarse and nodular lesion in histoplasmosis differentiate it from the fine reticular pattern seen with PCP.

c. The presence of lymphadenopathy distinguish histoplasmosis from PCP.

d. aspergillosis of lung is frequent in patients with HIV-induced immune deficiency

e. The most common chest radiographic manifestation of Cryptococcus neoformans is diffuse reticular opacification

39. Silo filler's disease refers to

a. obliterative bronchiolitis caused by Nitrogen dioxide

b. obliterative bronchiolitis caused by sulphur dioxide

c. obliterative bronchiolitis caused by ammonia

d. obliterative bronchiolitis caused by chlorine

e. obliterative bronchiolitis caused by phosgene

40.All are true regarding obliterative bronchiolitis except

a. irreversible circumferential submucosal fibrosis

b.absence of intraluminal granulation tissue polyps

c.no surrounding parenchymal inflammation

d.The epithelium overlying the abnormal fibrosis usually show ulceration

e. the accompanying artery is obliterated by fibrotic process in some cases

41.Lesions seen in Wegener's granulomatosis is/are all except

a. peripheral wedge-shaped lesions abutting the pleura mimicking pulmonary infarcts

b. a peribronchial distribution of consolidation

c. a region of focal consolidation with or without cavitation

d. always bilateral pleural effusions

e. Mild bronchiectasis

42.The most common manifestation of amiodarone-induced lung disease is

a.NSIP

b.diffuse alveolar damage

c.diffuse alveolar haemorrhage

d.organising pneumonia

e.eosinophilic pneumonia

43.The presence of irregular interfaces between the aerated lung parenchyma and bronchi,vessels or plerural surfaces is reffered as

a.sagging sign

b.the interface sign

c.beaded sign

d.spiculated sign

e.romantic sign

44.All are true of

peribronchovascular interstitial thickening except

a.appear as increase in bronchial wall thickening on HRCT

b.appear as an increase in diameter of pulmonary artery branches on HRCT

c.equivalent to peribronchial cuffing in chest x ray

d.smooth variety typical of lymphatic spread of carcinoma

e.nodular variety seen in pulmonary edema

45.All are direct sign of bronchiectasis except

a.Signet ring sign

b.string of sign

c.string of pearls

d.cluster of cysts

e.tubular or Y-shaped structures

46.All are true regarding pulmonary vascular disease except

a.dilatation of the main pulmonary artery indicates the presence of pulmonary hypertention

b.The main pulmonary artery measures up to 30 mm in diameter

c.The pulmonary artery to aortic diameter ratio of more than 2 strongly suggests pulmonary hypertention

d.mosaic perfusion refers to decreased lung attenuation with dcreased vessel size

e.enlargement of right ventricle and right atrium common in pulmonary hypertention

47.A elderly male with history of hypertention and hyperlipdemia

undergoes Cardiac MRI .All finding are consistent with myocardial infarction except

a.absent contractility

b.severely decreased perfusion

c.absent myocardial reserve

d.subendocardial enhancement on delayed scan

e.severely decreased myocardial stress perfusion

48.Modified Blalock–Taussig (BT) shunt for TOF refers to

a. the innominate artery and the left pulmonary artery

b. the innominate artery and the right pulmonary artery

c. the aorta and the right pulmonary artery

d. the aorta and the left pulmonary artery

e. the left pulmonary and the right pulmonary artery

49.The second most common cyanotic CHD in the first year of life

a. tetralogy of Fallot

b. transposition of great arteries (TGA).

c. common atria and common ventricles

d. PDA

e. persistent truncus arteriosus

50.All are true regarding Pneumocystis pneumonia except

a.caused by a fungus

b. Pneumatoceles is a late manifestation

c. Management of Spontaneous pneumothorax is notoriously difficult

d. Significant radiographic improvement is usually seen within 10 d of beginning treatment.
e. The radiographic appearance may get worse during the first 3 d of therapy

TEST PAPER 12 (ANSWER)

-

1---b
Calcification in empyema is most common in the lower posterior half of the chest. **(G)**

2-----e
The plain radiographic findings are of localized mesothelioma is a pleurally-based, well-demarcated, rounded and often slightly lobulated mass (2–20-cm diameter) which may, because of pedunculation, show marked positional variation with changes in posture and respiration.
Pleural fibromas usually make an obtuse angle with the chest wall . CT findings are similar to those observed on plain radiography: a mobile mass, often heterogeneous because of necrosis, haemorrhage, frequently enhancing after contrast medium administration, and rarely calcified.
Malignant types are usually larger than 10 cm and may invade the chest wall. Typically these tumours show low signal intensity on both T1- and T2-weighted images. **(G)**

3---c (Chapter 14,G)

4---e
Punctate foci of calcification may be seen. On CT the tumours may be homogeneous or heterogeneous, usually enhancing heterogeneously after intravenous contrast medium. (G)

5---e (Chapter 15, G)

6----e (Chapter 15, G)

7---b
CT, particularly HRCT, is the most accurate means of detecting emphysema and determining its type and extent in vivo. (Chapter 16, Large Airway Disease and chronic Airway Obstruction, Adam: Grainger & Allison's Diagnostic Radiology, 5th ed).

8----b
The most cost-effective and widely used method of screening for pulmonary metastases is CT scan. (Chapter 18, G)

9----c
Pleural effusion is common, seen in about 30% cases of lymphangitic carcinomatosis. (Chapter 18, G)

10---e (Chapter 18, G)

11---a
Lymphangioleiomyomatosis (LAM) is a rare disease seen almost exclusively in women, the vast majority of cases being diagnosed during childbearing age. LAM is a disease characterized histologically by two key features: cysts and proliferation of atypical smooth

muscle cells (LAM cells) of the pulmonary interstitium, particularly in the bronchioles, pulmonary vessels and lymphatics. (Chapter 19, G)

12---e (CHAPTER 22 ,G)
13---e (CHAPTER 22,G)
14---a (CHAPTER 23,G)
15---b (CHAPTER 23 ,G)
16---b (CHAPTER 24 ,G)
17---c (CHAPTER 24 ,G)
18---b

The arrangement in which the RCA reaches the crux of the heart and supplies the posterior descending artery occurs in about 85% and is termed right dominance. (CHAPTER 25,G)

19---e

Because atheroma is usually diffuse in the arterial wall, although not necessarily causing stenosis, arteriography tends to underestimate the degree of atheroma and the severity of the stenosis. (CHAPTER 25 ,G)

20---d

Approximately two-thirds of patients with pulmonary artery stenosis have additional cardiac lesions. (CHAPTER 6 .G)

21---e (CHAPTER 6 ,G)
22---e

Congenital inflammatory abnormalities that affect the aorta are Ehlers–Danlos and Marfan's syndromes, as well as neurofibromatosis. (CHAPTER 27,G)

23---c (CHAPTER 27 ,G)
24---b

Cystic congenital adenomatoid malformation and Diaphragmatic hernia cause mediastinal shift away from abnormal side. **(CHAPTER 64,G)**

25----a (CHAPTER 64,G)
26----d
27----c (Webb)
28----c

Gound glass opacity is due to morphological abnormalities below the resolution of HRCT and can reflect minimal thickening of the pulmonary interstitium or alveolar walls,presence of cells or fluid within the alveolar airspaces or an increase of in the capillary blood volume.(Webb)

29---e (CHAPTER 23 ,G)
30----b

The majority of patients with CCTGA have associated cardiac lesions, the most common being VSD. Pulmonary stenosis is present in approximately 50% of cases and tricuspid valve abnormalities (i.e. Ebstein's abnormality) are found in 20% of cases. (CHAPTER 23 ,G)

31---c

A right ventricle–pulmonary artery pathway is established in double outlet right ventricle —the Rastelli procedure.

Common arterial trunk (truncus arteriosus) is defined as a single arterial trunk arising from both ventricles, which overrides a large misaligned VSD. The pulmonary, systemic and coronary arteries originate from the single common arterial trunk..

In Type I, a short main pulmonary artery arises from the common trunk and subsequently divides. In Type II, the right and left pulmonary arteries originate from the posterior wall of the common trunkand in Type III, the right and left pulmonary arteries emerge from the lateral wall of the common trunk. (CHAPTER 23 .G)

32----d
In double outlet right ventricle , the Rastelli procedure is a method of surgical treatment. (CHAPTER 23 ,G)

33---e
Bilateral subpulmonary effusion doesnot cause bilateral symmetrical elevation of diaphragm.Elevation of diaphragm is mimicked by subpulmonary pleural effusion ,a large well-defined tumour adjacent to the dome or combined middle and lower lobe collapse .**(G)**

34----c
Disseminated lupus erythematosus cause bilateral elevation of dome of diaphragm. **(G)**

35---c (Chapter 14,G)

36----e
Aneurysms of the descending aorta appear as paravertebral mass ,other such lesions are he oesophageal or pharyngeal lesions (projecting posteriorly include leiomyoma, foregut duplication cyst, and congenital or acquireddiverticula of the oesophagus). The spinal origin of masses such as paraspinal abscess, primary or metastatic tumours of the vertebral body, or

haematoma from trauma to the spine are oviously paravertebral masses. (Chapter 14,G)

37----d
Cavitation is not expected in this setting. (Chapter 15, G)

38----d
Despite its importance as a complication of other immunosuppressive disorders, especially leukaemia and organ transplantation, aspergillosis is relatively infrequent in patients with HIV-induced immune deficiency. (Chapter 15,G)

39---a
Silo filler's disease refers to obliterative bronchiolitis caused by **Nitrogen dioxide.** (Chapter 16, G)

40---d
The epithelium overlying the abnormal fibrosis tissue may be flattened or metaplastic and is usually intact without any ulceration. (Chapter 16,G)

41---d
Unilateral or bilateral pleural effusions are present in about 10% of patients . (Chapter 19, G)

42---a (Chapter 19, G)
43-----b (Webb)
44----e
Pulmonary edema give rise to smooth peribronchovascular interstitial thickening.(Webb)
45-----e (Webb)
46----c
The pulmonary artery to aortic diameter ratio of more than 1

strongly suggests pulmonary hypertention

47-----d

There is either no defect or subendocardial enhancement on delayed scan in hibernating or stunned myocardium.There is a large transmural delayed enhancement in myocardial infarction.(Edelman)

48----b (CHAPTER 23 ,G)

49---b

Transposition of the great arteries (TGA) is the second most common cyanotic CHD in the first year of life with an incidence of 315 per million live births. (CHAPTER 23 ,G)

50----b

Pneumatoceles generally appear within a few days of the initial pneumonia, are thin walled, may rapidly increase or decrease in size, and over the course of 2–3 months gradually resolve
Significant radiographic improvement is usually seen within 10 d of beginning treatment. The radiographic appearance may get worse during the first 3 d of therapy, especially with intravenous trimethoprim–sulphamethoxazole, possibly related to overhydration pulmonary oedema and possibly to an inflammatory reaction to dead and dying parasites. (Chapter 15,G)

TEST PAPER 13

1.The only reliable indicator of chest wall invasion in bronchegenic carcinoma is
a. rib destruction
b.large contact (>3 cm) between the mass and the pleura,
c.an obtuse angle between the tumour and the chest wall,
d.an associated pleural thickening
e. the presence of pleural tags

2.All are true except
a. MRI has a slight advantage over CT in the evaluation of chest wall and pleura invasion
b. MRI showed higher sensitivity than spiral CT for superior sulcus tumour
c. spiral CT had higher specificity than MRI for superior sulcus tumour
d. CT is superior in the detection of pleural calcifications and osseous destruction
e. Pleural metastases are the most common pleural neoplasms

3.The most common extra-abdominal location of a neuroblastoma
a.anterior mediastinum
b.middle mediastinum
c.posterior mediastinum
d.brain
e.orbit

4.All are true regarding sympathetic ganglion tumour except

a. Ganglioneuromas are benign neoplasms usually occurring in children and young adults
b. Ganglioneuroblastomas exhibit variable degrees of malignancy and usually occur in children
c. Neuroblastomas are highly malignant tumours that typically occur in children younger than 5 years of age
d. Ganglioneuromas and ganglioneuroblastomas usually arise from the sympathetic ganglia in the posterior mediastinum
e. a horizontal orientation along the nerve

5.The most important (worldwide) pulmonary complication of HIV infection
a. tuberculosis
b. *Pneumocystis jiroveci (carinii)* pneumonia
c. community-acquired pneumonias
d. airways disease
e.kaposi sarcoma

6.Radiological features of Pneumocystis pneumonia are all except
a. bilateral, diffuse, symmetrical, fine to medium reticular opacities.
b. Pleural effusion very common
c. lymphadenopathy are rare
d. Pneumatoceles in 10% of patients
e. Spontaneous pneumothorax observed in approximately 5% of patients

7.True regarding emphysema are all except

a. Centrilobular emphysema shows predominance of upper lobe

b. mild paraseptal emphysema is very difficult to detected on HRCT

c. Panlobular emphysema is almost always most severe in the lower lobes

d. Panlobular emphysema(secondary to α_1-antitrypsin deficiency) is frequently associated with bronchiectasis.

e. areas of abnormally low attenuation associated with features of fibrosis is noted in irregular emphysema

8.All are true regarding bullae except

a. avascular

b. low-attenuation areas(>1 cm in diameter)

c. no wall

d. CT more sensitive than the chest radiograph in demonstrating bullae

e. CT useful for identifying patients suitable for treatment with bullectomy.

9.Miliary metastases are note most commonly in all except

a. thyroid

b.renal carcinomas

c.bone sarcomas

d. choriocarcinoma.

e.breast carcinoma

10.All are true regarding solitary pulmonary nodule except

a.size less than 3 cm

b. mostly benign

c. solitary circumscribed pulmonary opacity

d. no associated pulmonary, pleural, or mediastinal abnormality

e. Pleural tumours or plaques

11.All are true regarding cysts in Lymphangioleiomyomatosis (LAM)

a. numerous thin-walled cysts

b. zonal predilection

c. no sparing of the bases

d. more regularly shaped cysts

e. normal intervening lung parenchyma

12.All are true regarding rheumatoid arthritis except

a. pleuropulmonary disease may antedates the development of arthritis

b. in general, pleuropulmonary involvement is not related to the severity of the arthritis.

c. ILD in RA is more common in men with seropositive disease

d. The most common histopathological pattern in RA-associated ILD is NSIP

e. prognosis for RA–ILD is better than for idiopathic cases.

13. CTA is of proven accuracy and value in evaluating

a. great vessel anatomy (arterial and venous)

b.cardiac dimensions

c.ventricular function

d.viability,

e. perfusion and coronary artery anatomy

14.Correctly matched reconstruction methods is/are
a. Curved MPR --- evaluating the coronary arteries
b. Maximum intensity projection--contrast-enhanced 3D MRA as well as CTA
c. Surface shaded display-- for demonstrating the pulmonary veins using CTA or contrast-enhanced MRA
d. Volume rendered techniques---CTA or contrast-enhanced MRA, as well as imaging the airways, bowel and bone
e.all

15.All are features of situs solitus except
a. the IVC to the left of the abdominal aorta
b. The right-sided bronchus much shorter than the left-sided bronchus
c. heart on the left
d. stomach on the left
e. a right-sided liver

16.The best method of determining atrial identification is
a.size
b.shape
c.location
d.appendage
e.outlet/inlet

17.All are true regardind cardiac amyloidosis except
a. low compliance restrictive cardiomyopathy
b. decreased T1 of the myocardium
c. qualitative global and subendocardial delayed enhancement
d.good prognostic factor for amyloidosis

e. Familial amyloidosis due to the production of an unstable variant of the serum protein transerythretin (ATTR amyloidosis)

18.All are true regarding cardiomyopathy except
a. patchy areas of hyperenhancement in cardiac sarcoid
b. reduced tissue T1- and T2-relaxation rates in haemochromatosis
c. CMR of no use in monitoring treatment of haemochromatosis
d. Idiopathic volume-restricted cardiomyopathy mainly a disease of children
e. large ventricle with normal sized aria in Idiopathic volume-restricted cardiomyopathy

19.All are true regarding anastomosis in coronary artery obstruction except
a. The ring of Vieussens form anastomosis around the right ventricular conus
b. The ring of Vieussens is anastomosis between the LCA and the anterior descending artery
c. An anastomosis between an atrial branch and the atrioventricular nodal artery is called Kugel's artery
d. Septal anastomoses develop in the ventricular septum between branches of the anterior descending and posterior descending arteries
e. Septal anastomoses develop in the ventricular septum between atrial branches proximally and distally

20.All are true regarding coronary artery aneurysm except

164

a. Most aneurysms of the coronary arteries are congenital
b. Men are more commonly affected than women
c. False aneurysm may complicate PCI
d. seen in children in the mucocutaneous lymph node syndrome (Kawasaki disease)
e. often can be fully evaluated using CTA or CMR.

21.All are physiological changes of pulmonary embolism except
a. Arterial hypoxia
b. the development of alveolar dead space
c. pulmonary oedema
d. Lung volume reduction
e. pulmonary arterial hypotension

22.All are true regarding chest x-ray in pulmonary embolism except
a. normal in up to 40% of patients with PE
b. used to exclude other causes of the patient's symptoms (e.g. pneumothorax) rather than diagnosing PE
c. the overall sensitivity for diagnosis is high
d. often the first imaging examination requested
e. the overall specificity for the diagnosis is low

23.All are true regarding Granulomatous vasculitis (Takayasu's disease) except
a. The female-to-male ratio ---9:1 in Japan and 1.3:1 in India

b. the thoraco-abdominal aorta is mainly involved in patients from Korea and India
c. nodular fibrosis in all layers of the artery
d.common in Caucasians
e. The diagnosis depends on typical angiographic morphology

24. The angiographic features of the Granulomatous vasculitis (Takayasu's disease) include all except
a. luminal irregularity
b.vessel stenosis/ occlusion
c.dilatation
d. aneurysms
e.dissection

25.All are causes of paediatric lung cysts except
a. Bronchopulmonary sequestration (basal)
b. Cystic congenital adenomatoid malformation (basal cysts)
c. Kerosene inhalation
d. Histiocytosis
e.all

26.All are true of pulmonary venolobar syndrome except
a. theaffected lung lobe is normally connected to the bronchial tree
b. usually the right lower lobe affected
c. the abnormal vein draining the affected lobe drains to the left atrium.
d. a small ipsilateral lung with mediastinal shift towards the affected side

e. An abnormal vessel has shape of 'scimitar' sword

27.A farmer is recurrently exposed to moist hay .Initial presentation was that of fever ,chills,dry cough,dyspnea which lead to progressive shortness of breath later on.On the basis of history hypersensitivity pneumonitis was suspected .All are true regarding radiology of such case except

a.involvement of the lung bases in chronic cases

b.patchy or diffuse ground glass opacity

c.small il-defined centrilobular nodules

d.mosaic perfusion on expiratory scan

e.air trapping on expiratory scan

28. A patient is having fever cough ,weight loss shortness of breath for more than 3months and reveals peripheral eosinophilia on blood examination.All radiological features are consistent with diagnosis of chronic eosinophilic pneumonia except

a.peripheral airspace consolidation

b. predominant upper lobe distribution

c.photographic negative of the pulmonary edema

d.transient or fleeting pulmonary infiltrates

e.areas of consolidation unchanged over weeks or months

29.A young patients with smoking addiction has features of bone ,lung pituitary gland involvement .On suspicion of LCH,HRCT of lung was done .The finding suggestive of LCH are all except

a.bilateral lesions with predominance in upper and middle lung zones

b.relative sparing of costophrenic angles

c.thin-walled cyst,usually bizarre in shape

d.centrilobular and peribronchiolar nodules

e.decreased lung volumes

30.All are true except

a.nodules in LCH tend to be centrilobular

b.cysts in LCH is surrounded by abnormal parenchyma

c.centribobular emphysema may simulate LCH

d.upper lobe distribution of cyst in LCH

e.cysts in LCH may mimic the signet ring sign of bronchiectasis

31.All are true regarding Transposition of the great arteries (TGA) except

a. ventriculo-atrial discordance

b. an anterior aorta arise from the anterior right ventricle

c. the arterial switch operation the procedure of choice for TGA.

d. VSD in 40% of TGA cases

e. the Senning and Mustard procedure uses an intra-atrial baffle

32.The imaging modality of choice for pre-operative diagnosis and assessment of TGA

a. PET

b.chest x ray
c.MDCT
d. trans-thoracic echocardiography
e.MRI

33.All are true regarding mediastinal masses except

a. Almost all masses located superiorly in the anterior mediastinum causing focal deviation of the trachea are likely to be thyroid in origin.

b. Fat, fluid, or teeth within an anterior mediastinal mass are pathognomonic of cystic teratoma.

c. lymphangiomas show numerous areas of nonenhancing, water or near-water attenuation on CT

d. pericardial cysts has uniform water attenuation with a thin wall of uniform thickness and is in contact with the pericardium.

e. liposarcomas show homogenous CT attenuation value .

34.HRCT features of emphysema are all except

a. areas of abnormally low attenuation

b. distinct walls

c. multiple, small areas of emphysema scattered throughout the lung characteristic of centrilobular emphysema

d. paraseptal emphysema visible in the subpleural areas, along the peripheral or mediastinal pleura

e. widespread areas of abnormally low attenuation with paucity of vascular markings characteristic of panlobular emphysema

35.The most common and most important manifestation of AIDS in sub-saharan Africa is

a.tuberculosis

b. Pneumocystis jiroveci (formerly carinii)

c. Cryptococcus neoformans

d. Histoplasma capsulatum

e. Toxoplasma gondii

36.Worldwide, the most common cause of death among AIDS patients is

a.tuberculosis

b. Pneumocystis jiroveci (formerly carinii)

c. Cryptococcus neoformans

d. Histoplasma capsulatum

e. Toxoplasma gondii

37.All are true regarding role of computed tomography in assessing the distribution and severity of emphysema except

a. CT densitometry provides better correlation with a morphological reference than visually assed CT scores

b.In density mask technique, Pixels with values below a certain number(such as -950 HU) is highlighted on a CT image

c. the density mask method has been used as a means of distinguishing areas of simple hyperinflation without tissue destruction from areas of emphysema.

d. Expiratory CT does not correlate as well as inspiratory HRCT with the morphological extent of emphysema

e. the expiratory HRCT is inferior to inspiratory HRCT in reflecting functional air trapping

38.All are causes of obliterative bronchiolitis except
a. eruthromycin
b. Rheumatoid arthritis
c. Cystic fibrosis
d. Hypersensitivity pneumonitis
e. Sauropus androgynus ingestion

39.All are causes of solitary pulmonary nodule except
a. Bronchial carcinoma
b. Bronchial carcinoid
c. Granuloma
d. Hamartoma
e. Encysted pleural fluid

40.All are true regarding solitary pulmonary nodule except
a.dubling time of most peripheral pulmonary carcinomas is is more than 18 months
b. A lack of enhancement (< 15 HU) is indicative of benignity
c. ill-defined margins with umlication may be noted in carcinoma
d. PET or PET–CT has sensitivity, specificity and accuracy of 90% or greater in the diagnosis of benign nodules
e. False-negative results PET may occur in bronchiolo-alveolar carcinoma.

41.All are true regarding ventilation perfusion imaging except
a. negative examination can does not allow confident exclusion of the diagnosis of PE
b. Perfusion (Q) scintigraphy assess the distribution of pulmonary blood flow
c. Ventilation (V) scintigraphy is performed by inhalation of krypton-81m, xenon-133
d. Matched ventilation and perfusion defects are commonly seen in patient with obstructive airways disease
e. provides a probability assessment of the risk of the presence of a PE

42.Shrinking lung syndrome is noted in
a.SLE
b.Rheumatoid arthritis
c.Sjogren syndrome
d. Polymyositis (PM)
e.Tuberculosis

43.All are causes of bilateral upper lobe fibrosis except
a. Tuberculosis
b. Sarcoidosis
c. Allergic bronchopulmonary aspergillosis
d. Chronic extrinsic allergic alveolitis
e.SLE

44.The most common lung imaging finding in Wegener's granulomatosis is
a. fibrosing lung disease
b. Multiple nodules or masses
c. Airspace consolidation
d. ground-glass opacities
e. pleural effusions

45.Limitation of Coronary computed tomography angiography

a. imaging of vessels smaller than 6 mm

b. imaging of vessels smaller than 5 mm

c. imaging of vessels smaller than 2 mm

d. imaging of vessels smaller than 4 mm

e. imaging of vessels smaller than 3 mm

46..All are correctly matched sequence except

a. black blood imaging (spin-echo, turbo spin-echo) is used for anatomical imaging

b. cine-MRA (white blood imaging) is used to assess dynamic function

c. Phase-contrast imaging is used to measure blood flow velocity

d. Contrast enhancement can be used for extracardiac angiography using 3D gradient-echo sequences

e. FLAIR sequences can be used to identify areas of myocardial injury

47. Right isomerism is characterized by all except

a. bilateral (short) right bronchi

b. trilobed lungs

c. bilateral right atrial appendages

d.polysplenia

e. a midline liver.

48. Left isomerism is usually associated all except

a. bilateral left (long) bronchi

b.bilobed lungs

c.left atrial appendages

d.polysplenia

e.IVC continuation

49.All are true regarding endomyocardial fibrosis (EMF)

a. predominantly affects the peoples of equatorial Africa, southern India, Sri Lanka, and Brazil

b. deposition of a layer of fibrous tissue on the ventricular endocardium

c. In non-caucasians, the pathological process usually involves the right heart

d. fibrous tissue deposition beginning at the AV valve

e. Very rarely curvilinear calcification due to endocardial calcification

50.All are true regarding left ventricular noncompaction except

a. form of congenital cardiomyopathy

b. myocardium (more often the left ventricle) has a 'spongy' appearance

c. trabeculations in the ventricular apex on echo

d. the presence of two myocardial layers with different degrees of tissue compaction on CMR

e. sporadic in nature

TEST PAPER 13 (ANSWER)

1---a
Features such as a large contact (>3 cm) between the mass and the pleura, an obtuse angle between the tumour and the chest wall, an associated pleural thickening and the presence of pleural tags are usually considered as signs of chest wall invasion ,but they also occur in benign lesions. The only reliable indicator is rib destruction. **(G)**

2----b
Spiral CT and MRI showed comparable sensitivity for superior sulcus tumour.**(G)**

3----c
The most common extra-abdominal location of a neuroblastoma is posterior mediastinum (Chapter 14, G)

4----e
Ganglioneuromas and ganglioneuroblastomas usually arise from the sympathetic ganglia in the posterior mediastinum and therefore usually present radiologically as well-defined elliptical masses, with a vertical orientation, extending over the anterolateral aspect of three to five vertebral bodies. Neuroblastomas are typically more heterogeneous due to areas of haemorrhage, necrosis, cystic degeneration and calcium. They may be locally invasive and have a tendency to cross the midline. (Chapter 14, G)

5---a (Chapter 15,G)

6---b
Pleural fluid and lymphadenopathy are rare or do not occur unless extrapulmonary involvement has been observed, usually in patients who have received prophylactic aerosolized pentamidine.
Unusual radiographic presentations include diffuse or focal miliary nodules, homogeneous opacities, solitary or multiple well formed nodules and moderate to thick-walled cavitary nodules (Chapter 15, G)

7----b
Irregular emphysema is recognized on HRCT as areas of abnormally low attenuation associated with features of fibrosis. (Chapter 16,G)

8---c
Bullae are seen as avascular, low-attenuation areas that are larger than 1 cm in diameter and that can have a thin but perceptible wall. (Chapter 16,G)

9----e (Chapter 18, G)

10----e
Pleural tumours or plaques is a stimulant of a solitary pulmonary nodule (Chapter 18, G)

11-----b

The CT manifestations of LAM are distinctive, characterized by numerous thin-walled cysts randomly distributed throughout the lungs with no zonal predilection. Imaging features that help distinguish LAM from LCH include a more diffuse distribution of cysts typically with no sparing of the bases, more regularly shaped cysts and normal intervening lung parenchyma. (Chapter 19, G)

12----d

The most common histopathological pattern in RA-associated ILD is UIP. Pleral effusion is common.Other pulmonary abnormalities seen in RA include follicular bronchiolitis, bronchiectasis , obliterative bronchiolitis , methotrexate-induced pneumonitis and organizing pneumonia. (Chapter 19,G)

13---a

CTA is of proven accuracy and value in evaluating great vessel anatomy (arterial and venous). (CHAPTER 22 ,G)

14----e (CHAPTER 22,G)

15---a (CHAPTER 23 ,G)

16---d

The atrial appendages are the best method of determining atrial identification. The right atrial appendage is triangular with a wide base, whilst the left atrial appendage is a tubular structure.

The presence of the terminal crest and pectinate muscle in the appendage are more specific internal characteristics of the right atrium and its appendage. (CHAPTER 23 ,G)

17---d

Cardiac involvement in amyloidosis indicates a poor prognosis and also predicts poor tolerance to high dose chemotherapy and stem cell transplantation. (CHAPTER 24 ,G)

18----e

Large atria with normal sized ventricles is noted in Idiopathic volume-restricted cardiomyopathy. CHAPTER 24 ,G)

19---b

The ring of Vieussens is anastomosis between the RCA and the anterior descending artery. (CHAPTER 25,G)

20---a

Most aneurysms of the coronary arteries are atheromatous in nature,not congenital. (CHAPTER 25,G)

21---e

Pulmonary embolism cause pulmonary arterial hypertension .It is estimated that greater than 50% of the vasculature needs to be obstructed for there to be a significant rise in pulmonary arterial pressure. (CHAPTER 6,G)

22---c

The overall sensitivity and specificity of chest radiography for the diagnosis is low .In light of these findings the purpose of chest radiography is probably best thought of as one of excluding other causes of the patient's symptoms (e.g. pneumothorax) rather than diagnosing PE. (CHAPTER 6 ,G)

23----d

Racial variation occurs, the disease being uncommon in caucasians and affecting Sephardic Jews but not Ashkenazi Jews. The pattern of vessel involvement also varies in different parts of the world. The involvement of the aortic arch and its branches is common in Japan, whereas the thoraco-abdominal aorta is mainly involved in patients from Korea and India. (CHAPTER 27,G)

24----e (CHAPTER 27,G)

25----e (CHAPTER 64 ,G)

26---c

The vein draining the lobe (usually the right lower lobe) drains into the inferior vena cava or portal vein, rather than to the left atrium. An abnormal vessel is usually seen draining down and enlarging towards the diaphragm in the shape of a 'scimitar' sword. **(CHAPTER 64,G)**

27---a

Relative sparing of lung bases in chronic cases allows distinction of this entity from IPF ,in which fibrosis usually predominates in the lung bases.DIP and NSIP often have a subpleural predominance of areas of gound glass opacity and are rarely associated with centrilobular nodules.Alveolar opacity shows a crazy-paving appearance.(Webb)

28----d

Peripheral airspace onsolidation is noted in BOOP also but often onvolves the upper zone to a greater degree. Transient or fleeting pulmonary infiltrates is noted in simple pulmonary eosinophilia.(Webb)

29----e

Lung volumes are characteristically normal or increased.(Webb)

30---b

Cysts in LCH is surrounded by normal parenchyma .(Webb)

31----a

Transposition of the great arteries (TGA) is defined as ventriculo-arterial discordance with an anterior aorta arising from the anterior right ventricle, and the pulmonary artery arising from the posterior left ventricle. In the Senning and Mustard procedure blood is diverted by an intra-atrial baffle from the right atrium to the left ventricle, and from the left atrium to the right ventricle. In arterial switch operation , the aorta and main pulmonary artery are transected just above the origin of the coronary arteries, switched and re-anastomosed to the correct ventricle. (CHAPTER 23 ,G)

32---d (CHAPTER 23 ,G)

33---e

Liposarcomas show an unusual mixture of fat interspersed by

irregular strands or masses of soft tissue attenuation. (Chapter 14,G)

34----b

Focal areas of emphysema usually lack distinct walls as opposed to lung cysts. (Chapter 16,G)

35----a (Chapter 15,G)

36---a (Chapter 15,G)

37----e

The expiratory HRCT is superior to inspiratory HRCT in reflecting functional air trapping. . (Chapter 16,G)

38----a (Chapter 16,G)

39----e (Chapter 18, G)

.

40----a

Benign lesions almost invariably have a doubling time of less than 1 month or more than 18 months, with the volume doubling time for most peripheral pulmonary carcinomas being between 1 and 18 months (median 3 months). Bronchiolo-alveolar carcinomas may grow slowly, with volume doubling times much longer than those usually quoted for bronchial carcinoma. (Chapter 18,G)

41.---a

Negative examination of ventilation perfusion imaging can allow confident exclusion of the diagnosis of PE. (CHAPTER 6,G)

42----a (Chapter 19,G)

43---e

Other causes of bilateral upper lobe fibrosis are Histoplasmosis,

Ankylosing spondylitis, Progressive massive fibrosis (distinctive mass-like opacities). (Chapter 19, G)

44----b

Multiple nodules or masses are the most common imaging finding in Wegener's granulomatosis(70%).Nodules range in size from a few millimetres to 10 cm, are frequently multiple, and increase in size and number as the disease progresses. Nodules are bilateral in 75% of cases, have no predilection for any lung zone, and usually show cavitation at about 2 cm in size. (Chapter 19,G)

45---c

Heavy calcification, which may prevent visualization of the artery lumen and imaging of vessels smaller than 2 mm are limitations of Coronary computed tomography angiography. (CHAPTER 22 ,G)

46----e

Inversion recovery type sequences (with or without contrast medium injection) can be used to identify areas of myocardial injury. . (CHAPTER 22,G)

47----d

Right isomerism is characterized by asplenia. (CHAPTER 23,G)

48----e

Left isomerism is usually associated with bilateral left (long) bronchi, bilobed lungs, left atrial appendages, polysplenia and IVC interruption. (CHAPTER 23 ,G)

49---d

Endomyocardial fibrosis (EMF) is characterized by the deposition of a layer of fibrous tissue on the ventricular endocardium, beginning at the apex and spreading proximally to encroach on the atrioventricular valve. CHAPTER 24 ,G)

50---e

Left ventricular noncompaction (LVNC) is a rare form of congenital cardiomyopathy and is often familial. CHAPTER 24 ,G)

TEST PAPER 14

1.True about acinus
a) 0.5–0.6 mm in diameter,
b) comprises alveolar ducts and alveoli only
c) secondary pulmonary lobule comprises thirty to fifty acini
d) peripheral interlobular septa give rise to septal or Kerley A lines
e) comprises respiratory bronchioles, alveolar ducts and alveoli.

2. All are true regarding pulmonary anatomy except
a) the respiratory bronchioles are the last purely conducting airways
b) the pores of Kohn link different alveolar units
c) the secondary pulmonary lobule is the smallest unit of lung bounded by connective tissue septa
d) the secondary pulmonary lobule is best seen sub-pleurally
e) the centrilobular arteries can be resolved HRCT in the normal lung

3. Poland syndrome is characterized by all except
a) Unilateral absence or hypoplasia of the pectoralis major.
b) contraleral hand and arm anomalies (particularly syndactyly)
c) ipsilateral absence of pectoralis minor,
d) ipsilateral rib anomalies,

e) ipsilateral hypoplasia of breast and nipple.

4.all are true regarding soft tissue tumour of chest wall except
a) the most common primary benign tumour is neurofibroma
b) the most common primary malignant tumour is lipo/fibrosarcoma
c) neurofibromas have a lower density than muscle both in pre and post contrast (CT)
d) neurofibromas give low to intermediate signal on T1W, high signal on T2W and shows marked contrast enhancement
e) Lymphangiomas on CT have the features of a fluid-filled cyst with or without septation

5.All are true regarding percentage of mediastinal masses in adult surgical series except
a) neuroblastoma/ganglioneuroma(10%)
b) thymic (20–25%) origin
c) neoplasm of lymph nodes (10–20%).
d) Developmental cysts(10%)
e) neurogenic (17–23%)

6.The most useful imaging investigation for localizing, characterizing and

demonstrating the extent of a
mediastinal mass and its
relationship to adjacent
structures is
a) CT
b) MRI
c) ULTRASOUND
d) PET-CT
e) Radionuclide

**7.All are true regarding lobar
pneumonia except**
a)usually unifocal
b)develops in the distal airspaces
c) uniform homogeneous
opacification
d)the airways primarily involved
e.air bronchograms common

**8.All are true regarding
bronchopneumonia except**
a) frequently caused by aspiration
b) usually multifocal
c) centred in distal airways.
d) initially characterized by large
heterogeneous, scattered opacities
e) an air bronchogram a constant
feature.

**9.All are true regarding trachea
except**
a) principal sites of stenosis   are at
the stoma or at the level of the
endotracheal or tracheostomy tube
balloon.
b)The most common primary
malignant neoplasms are
squamous cell carcinoma and
adenoid cystic carcinoma
c)The most common benign
neoplasms are hamartoma,
leiomyoma, neurogenic tumour and
lipoma
d)Involvement of the large airways
is a uncommon manifestation of
Wegener's granulomatosis

e) Symmetrical subglottic stenosis
is the most frequent manifestation
of relapsing polychontritis in chest

**.10.All are true regarding sabre-
sheath trachea except**
a) a diffuse narrowing of the
intrathoracic trachea
b) almost always associated with
COPD
c) the internal side-to-side diameter
of the trachea is more than the
corresponding sagittal diameter
d) an abrupt return to normal
calibre at the thoracic inlet
e) usually shows a smooth inner
margin

**11.All are true regarding causes
of lobar collapse except**
a) the frequent causes of intrinsic
obstruction in adults are tumours
and mucus plugs
b) lobar collapse should always be
suspected to be due to a
bronchogenic carcinoma in elderly
smoker until proved otherwise
c) inhaled foreign bodies /mucus
plugs in children are common
causes of lobar collapse
d) tumours is   a common cause of
lobar collapse in children
e) bronchiolo-alveolar cell
carcinoma may cause lobar
collapse without endobronchial
obstruction

**12.All are true regarding
radiographic features of lung
collapse except**
a) increased opacity of the affected
lobe
b) volume loss
c) displacement of interlobar
fissures

d) spreading of pulmonary vessels and bronchi

e) hyperinflation of other lobes

13.All are true regarding lung collapse except

a) upper lobe collapse often results in a shift of the superior mediastinum

b) lower lobe collapse often demonstrates elevation of the diaphragm

c) hilar elevation is a sign of upper lobe collapse

d) ipsilateral main bronchus becomes more vertcally orientated than usual with significant upper lobe collapse

e) displacement of the anterior junctional line to the contralateral side of large collapse

14.All are true regarding risk factors of bronchial carcinoma except

a) smoking increases risk of carcinoma 2-3 fold

b) exposure asbestos, nickel and arsenic

c) interstitial pulmonary fibrosis

d) radiotherapy.

e) smoking most important factor

15.The incidence of which lung carcinoma is decreasing

a) adenocarcinoma

b) squamous cell carcinoma

c) bronchiolo-alveolar carcinoma

d) large cell carcinoma

e) small cell carcinoma

16.All are true regarding interstitial lung disease except

a) HRCT provides insight into disease reversibility and prognosis.

b) a reticular pattern on CT almost always represents significant ILD

c) smooth Interlobular septal thickening is seen in pulmonary oedema

d) irregular interlobular septal thickening is seen in alveolar proteinosis

e) intralobular septal thickening seen in all ILDs

17.All are true regarding reticular pattern except

a) due to intelobular or intralobular thickening

b) subtle interlobular thickening may cause ground glass opacity

c) honeycomb lung has cystic spaces surrounded by irregular walls

d) may produce bronchiectasis/bronchiolectasis

e) Intralobular septal thickening is most commonly noted in IPF

18.All are true regarding rib fractures except

a) fractures of the 1st to 3rd ribs is common in trivial trauma

b) fractures in posterior aspects of rib in children should raise the possibility of nonaccidental injury

c) More than 50% of acute fractures are missed on initial radiographs

d) double fractures of three or more adjacent ribs are referred as 'flail chest'

e) rib fractures are usually of the greenstick variety in children

19.An abnormally deep costophrenic sulcus sign is noted in

a) pneumothorax in supine position
b) pleural effusion in supine position
c) pleural effusion in decubitus position
d) pneumothorax in standing position
e) collapse of lower lobe

20. All are true regarding airspace diseases except
a) Wegener's granulomatosis may show cavitation on CT scan
b) areas of consolidation in cryptogenic organizing pneumonia is most pronounced in the periphery and lower zones of the lungs
c) changes in chronic eosinophilic pneumonia tend to be in the upper zones and parallel to the chest wall
d) transient and migratory opacities with no significant constitutional disturbance favour diagnosis of an eosinophilic pneumonia.
e) 'crazy-paving' pattern on CT is noted in alveolar proteinosis.

21. All are true regarding central airways except
a) Lower limit of the mean transverse diameter is 12.3 mm for women and 15.9 mm for men
b) Calcification of the cartilage rings of the trachea is a common normal finding after the age of 40 years
c) volumetric thin-collimation CT can routinely identify airways to sub-segmental level
d) in the adult ,left main stem bronchus has a steeper angle than the right
e) The left main bronchus extends up to twice as far as the right main

bronchus before giving off its upper lobe division.

22. All are true regarding anatomy of right heart cavities except
a) the membranous septum lying above the tricuspid valve separates the left ventricle from the right atrium
b) the coronary sinus is the main draining vein of the heart
c) coronary sinus enter into the right atrium between the inferior vena cava and the pulmonary valve
d) the right coronary artery run in the anterior atrioventricular groove
e) infundibulum separates the right ventricular inflow and outflow

23. All are true regarding anatomy of left ventricles except
a) left ventricle is carrot-shaped
b) the membranous septum lies between the right and noncoronary sinuses of Valsalva
c) the membranous septum provides the right attachment to the posterior leaflet of the mitral valve
d) the smooth muscular septum curves round the upper part of the left ventricle,
e) the smooth muscular septum forms part of the left border of the left ventricle

24. All are direct sign of bronchiectasis on HRCT except
a) internal diameter of bronchi more than adjacent pulmonary artery
b) visibility of peripheral airways within 1 cm of the costal pleura
c) touching of the mediastinal pleura of peripheral airways
d) Lack of tapering of bronchi

greater than 2 cm distal to bifurcation

e) bronchial wall thickening

25.The fetal heart is most susceptible to rubella virus/thalidomide during

a) 2-3 week of intrauterine life

b) 3-5week of intrauterine life

c) 5-7week of intrauterine life

d) 7-9 week of intrauterine life

e) 9-11week of intrauterine life

26.Which is not a endocardial cushions defect

a) Ostium primum defect /Tricuspid atresia

b) Endocardial atrioventricular defect

c) Ostium secundum defect

d) Cor triatrium

e) Ebstein's anomaly

27.Cardiothoracic ratio for diagnosing cardiomegaly on PA view of chest x-ray in adult is

a) >40%

b) >45%

c) >50%

d) >55%

e) >60%

28.All are causes of mitral regurgitation except

a) Marfan's syndrome

b) mucopolysaccharidosis

c) systemic lupus erythematosis

d) rheumatoid arthritis

e) restrictive cardiomyopathy

29.The Agatston calcium score is related to

a) coronary calcification

b) pulmonary calcification

c) aortic calcification

d) renal calcification

e) carotid calcification

30.All are true regarding pulmonary circulation except

a) hypoxia causes arterial dilatation

b) both pulmonary and bronchial circulations supply the lung

c) the main pulmonary artery in adult measures approximately 5 cm in length

d) the main pulmonary artery is entirely enveloped within the pericardium

e) the main pulmonary artery divides to form the left and right pulmonary arteries at T4 vertebrae.

31.All are true regarding pulmonary artery except

a) left pulmonary artery arches superiorly over the left main bronchus

b) right pulmonary traverses the mediastinum posterior to the right main bronchus

c) The right pulmonary artery arises at a right angle from the main pulmonary trunk

d) The descending trunk passes vertically inferiorly from the right hilum

e) right pulmonary artery divides into the ascending and descending trunks just before entering the hilum

32.All are true regarding the normal aorta except

a) The aortic root is approximately 3 cm in diameter

b) The abdominal aorta is approximately 2 cm in diameter

c) The aortic root and most of the ascending aorta is contained within the pericardium
d) The ascending aorta does not form the mediastinal border on a PA chest radiograph
e) the descending thoracic aorta normally begins immediately beyond the origin of the left subclavian artery

33.All are true except
a) the innominate and left common carotid arteries have a common origin in 20% population
b) the left vertebral artery arises directly from the aortic arch in 6%
c) ligamentum venosum (the embryological ductus arteriosus) closes within a few days of birth
d) the aorta is fixed at point of attachment of ligmentum venosum
e) aorta arches over the root of the right lung

34.All are true regarding intervention except
a) Angioplasty refers to treatment of a vascular stenosis or occlusion with a balloon catheter
b) Stenting refers to the placement of a metallic mesh tube across a vascular stenosis or occlusion
c) balloon expandable endoprostheses are mounted on a balloon catheter and deployed by deflating the balloon
d) self-expanding stents are compressed on a delivery catheter and released by withdrawing an outer sheath
e) embolization refers to the occlusion of a blood vessel by injection of embolic material

through a catheter

35----669.All are embolic agents except
a) metallic springs (coils) and particulate matter
b) gelatin sponge
c) glue
d) absolute alcohol
e) all

36.All of the following are true regarding neonatal chest except
a) almost cylindrical in shape
b) The ribs have a less horizontal orientation
c) level of the diaphragm at the sixth to eighth anterior rib
d) The normal cardiothoracic ratio can be as large as 65% due to the presence of the thymus
e) sternal ossification centres may simulate healing rib fractures

37.All are true regarding thymus except
a) the presence of the thymus may increase normal cardiothoracic ratio.
b) the size of the thymus can be highly variable.
c) a normal thymus does not compress or displace other structures
d) the thymus may involute rapidly in association with prenatal or postnatal stress
e) the thymus may rapidly increase following the administration of exogenous steroids

38.All are true regarding radiological evaluation of tubes and lines except

a) optimal positioning for an endotracheal tube (ETT) is approximately 1–1.5 cm above the carina

b) the umbilical arterial line lies just lateral to the right side of the spine.

c) the tip of umbilical arterial line should ideally lie between T6 and T10 to avoid the spinal artery

d) the tip of umbilical arterial line should ideally lie at L3–L5 below the level of the bowel and renal arteries

e) the umbilical vein catheter tip lies above the liver and has not passed into a tributary vein

39. A 10 year old child suffering from parasitic infection with minimal symptoms shows peripheral blood eosinophilia .X ray shows transient bilateral airspace opacification which resolves within a week.Which of following is the most likely diagnosis

a) Simple pulmonary eosinophilia (Löffler's syndrome)

b) Acute eosinophilic pneumonia

c) Chronic eosinophilic pneumonia

d) Wegener's granulomatosis

e) Hypereosinophilic syndrome

40.A male patients (30 yrs)presented with exertional dyspnoea and non-productive cough and showed evidence of digital clubbing and inspiratory

crackes.X ray showed bilateral airspace opcification pronounced in central area.The broncho-alveolar lavage revealed periodic acid-Schiff-positive lipoproteinaceous material .What is the expected chararacheristic HRCT finding is this case?

a) miliary lesions

b) honeycombing

c) crazy-paving pattern

d) diffuse emphysema

e) multiple holes

41.Up to two-thirds of myocardial infarctions are caused

a) by plaque rupture on a nonobstructive (<50%) lesion

b) by plaque rupture on a obstructive (>60%) lesion

c) by plaque rupture on a normal caliber artery

d) by calcium deposit on a nonobstructive (<50%) lesion

e) by calcium deposit on a obstructive (>60%) lesion

42.A cardiac patient on amiodarone and amlodipine therapy is subjected to CT scan of chest which shows high attenuation nodules ,the most likely cause is

a) amiodarone toxicity

b) microlithiasis

c) metastatic calcification

d) tuberculosis

e) amlodipine

43.All are true except

a) honeycombing has clearly

definable wall (1-3mm thick)
b) LIP does not show cysts
c) cyst in LAM and LCH donot share wall
d) honeycombing occur in several layers
e) pneumatoceles seen in pneumonia

44. Features of asbestosis are usually most severe in
a) the subpleural regions of the lower lobes
b) centre of lower lobes
c) the subpleural regions of the upper lobes
d) the subpleural regions of the mid lobes
e) the central regions of the upper lobes

45.All are true regarding inflammatory abdominal aortic aneurysm (IAAA) except
a) the ureters can be involved in the inflammatory process
b) duodenum and left renal vein are often adherent to the aneurysm sac
c) IAAA repair halts the progression of retroperitoneal fibrosis but does not cure it
d) In peri-aortitis, CT shows a thick cuff of non -enhancing soft tissue around the aorta
e) endovascular aneurysm repair is an attractive option for treatment

46. Intermediate probability studies or a low probability study of V/Q scan with strong clinical suspicion has pulmonary embolism in what percentage of cases
a) up to 40%

b) up to 60%
c) up to 80%
d) up to 20%
e) up to 10%

47.Ancillary signs of pulmonary embolism are all except
a) intravascular filling defect and a 'tram track' appearance
b) small pleural effusions
c) focal infarcts in the costophrenic recesses
d) enlargement of the bronchial vessels
e) prominent mosaic attenuation pattern

48.All are true regarding VSDs except
a) Perimembranous lesions account for 80% of all VSDs
b) initial assessment with echocardiography
c) most of perimembranous VSDs donot close spontaneously
d) 'Swiss cheese appearance' noted in muscular VSD
e) an associated additional cardiac abnormality rare

49.All are true regarding Eisenmenger syndrome except
a) noted in left-to-right shunt
b) high pulmonary vascular resistance
c) tends to occur earlier in life in VSD and patent ductus
d) the large central pulmonary arteries
e) The increasing prevalence of Eisenmenger syndrome

50.All are true regarding cardiac imaging except
a) SPECT imaging shows sensitivity of 91% and specificity

of 89% in diagnosis of coronary artery disease (chronic chest pain)
b) a normal perfusion scintigraphy does not excludes acute infarction
c) myocardial perfusion imaging is a better indicator of prognosis than clinical assessment, exercise ECG, or coronary angiography
d) left ventricular ejection fraction (LVEF) at the time of discharge or 10–14 d after infarction predicts mortality
e) radionuclide ventriculography is standard practice for patients receiving cardiotoxic chemotherapy such as doxorubicin

TEST PAPER 14 (ANSWER)

1.---- e

Acinus (5–6 mm in diameter) comprises respiratory bronchioles, alveolar ducts and alveoli. Secondary pulmonary lobule comprises three to five acini .Peripheral interlobular septa on thickening give rise to septal or Kerley B lines.(G)

2.----a

The terminal bronchioles are the last purely conducting airways of the bronchial tree and the region of lung subtended by a terminal bronchiole is termed the acinus (comprising the respiratory bronchioles, alveolar ducts, alveolar sacs and alveoli). The centrilobular arteries (with a diameter of 0.2 mm) can be resolved on high-resolution computed tomography (HRCT) in the normal lung, whereas normal bronchioles with a diameter below 2 mm are generally not seen. The secondary pulmonary lobule is best seen sub-pleurally, measuring between 5 and 30 incorporating 3–24 acini.Infiltration of the interlobular interstitium by oedema fluid or malignant cells, or thickening by fibrosis, will render individual secondary pulmonary lobules visible on HRCT. (G)

3.-----b

Unilateral absence or hypoplasia of the pectoralis major results in a unilateral transradiancy and an abnormal anterior axillary fold in Poland's syndrome. These changes are accompanied by ipsilateral hand and arm anomalies (particularly syndactyly) with or without absence of pectoralis minor,

rib anomalies, and hypoplasia of breast and nipple. (G)

4.----a

The most common primary benign tumour of soft tissue of chest wall is lipoma (G)

5.-----a

In adult surgical series, the most frequent tumours are of neurogenic (17–23%) or thymic (20–25%) origin, or are neoplastic disorders of lymph nodes (10–20%). Developmental cysts, thyroid masses, and germ-cell tumours constitute the next most frequent group (approximately 10% each).In children, neuroblastoma/ganglioneuroma, foregut cysts and germ-cell tumours account for over three-quarters of cases, whereas thymoma and thyroid masses are rare. (G)

6.-----a

Computed tomography is the most useful investigation for localizing, characterizing and demonstrating the extent of a mediastinal mass and its relationship to adjacent structures.Magnetic resonance imaging remains useful for imaging suspected neurogenic tumours, for demonstrating intraspinal extension of a mediastinal mass and for further evaluating the relationship of a mass to the heart, pericardium and larger intrathoracic vessels. (G)

7.----d
In lobar pneumonia, the airways are not primarily involved and remain patent, there is little to no volume loss and air bronchograms are common. (G)

8.-----e
An air bronchogram is usually absent in bronchopneumonia. (G)

9.-----d
Involvement of the large airways is a common manifestation of Wegener's granulomatosis. (G)

10.----c
The internal side-to-side diameter of the trachea is halved or less than the corresponding sagittal diameter in sabre-sheath trachea.(G)

11.----d
In children, tumours is a very rare cause of lobar collapse .(G)

12.-----d
The pulmonary vessels and bronchi become crowded together in the affected lobe as the lung loses volume. (G)

13.----d
In significant upper lobe collapse, the ipsilateral main bronchus

becomes more horizontally orientated than usual, hence the bronchus intermedius and the left lower lobe bronchus swing laterally. In case of lower lobe collapse, each main bronchus is more vertically orientated than usual, with a medial swing of the bronchus intermedius on the right and the lower lobe bronchus on the left. (G)

14-----a
Tobacco smoke is the most important causative agent imparting a 20–30-fold increased risk in smokers compared to non-smokers. (G)

15-----b (G)

16.----d
Interlobular septal thickening is usually described as smooth (seen in pulmonary oedema and alveolar proteinosis) or irregular (lymphangitic spread of tumour). Intralobular septal thickening manifests as a fine reticular pattern on HRCT and is seen in all ILDs but most commonly in IPF. (G)

17----b
The intralobular septal thickening may be so fine that HRCT does not demonstrate discrete intralobular opacities but a generalized increase in lung density (ground-glass opacification). (G)

18.----a
Fractures of the 1st to 3rd ribs imply severe trauma.(G)

19.----a
With supine radiographs, air collects anterior to the lung and

there is no visible lung edge. In this situation a pneumothorax can produce an unusually sharp mediastinal border and hemidiaphragm and an abnormally deep costophrenic sulcus.(G)

20.----b

Areas of consolidation in cryptogenic organizing pneumonia are most pronounced in the periphery and upper zones of the lungs. (G)

21.----d

In adults, the right main stem bronchus has a steeper angle than the left.(G)

22.-----c

Coronary sinus enter into the right atrium between the inferior vena cava and the tricuspid valve . (G)

23.----c

The membranous septum provides the right attachment to the anterior leaflet of the mitral valve. (G)

24.---e

Bronchial wall thickening is indirect sign of bronchiestasis.(Webb)

25.-----b

The fetal heart develops between the second (total fetal length 2 mm) and eighth week of intrauterine life. It is during the third to fifth weeks of intrauterine life (when the forelimbs are developing) that the cardiac structures develop most actively and are therefore most susceptible to adverse external influence (e.g. rubella virus or drugs such as thalidomide). (G)

26.-----c. (G)

27.----c (G)

28.----e

Hypertrophic cardiomyopathy causes mitral regurgitation.(G)

29.----a (G)

30.----a

The pulmonary circulation's response to hypoxia is arterial constriction. (G)

31.----b

The right pulmonary artery arises at a right angle from the main pulmonary trunk, traverses the mediastinum posterior to the superior vena cava and ascending aorta and anterior to the right main bronchus, and just before entering the hilum it divides into the ascending and descending trunks.(CHAPTER 26 ,G)

32.---d

Ascending aorta forms the right mediastinal border on a postero-anterior (PA) chest radiograph. (CHAPTER 27,G)

33.-----e

A normal aorta passes superiorly and to the right for approximately 5 cm, then arches posteriorly and to the left over the root of the left lung. (CHAPTER 27,G)

34.-----c

Balloon expandable endoprostheses are mounted on a balloon catheter and deployed by inflating the balloon. (CHAPTER 28,G)

35.-----e (CHAPTER 28 ,G)

36.----b

On a rotated chest radiograph sternal ossification centres may simulate healing rib fractures or lung opacities . The ribs have a more horizontal orientation.

(CHAPTER 64.G)

37.-----e

The thymus may involute rapidly in association with prenatal or postnatal stress or following the administration of exogenous steroids. **(CHAPTER 64 .G)**

38.----b

The umbilical arterial line initially courses caudally through the internal and common iliac arteries to enter the aorta, and lies just lateral to the left side of the spine. The umbilical vein catheter courses directly cephalad on the right side of the abdomen and enters the left portal vein, at which point it may enter the ductus venosus and then the inferior vena cava. Radiographs should confirm that the tip lies above the liver and has not passed into a tributary vein **(CHAPTER 64,G)**

39.----a

The airspace opacification in Löffler's syndrome is fleeting and may be either uni- or bi-lateral. Resolution of opacities within a period of days and, by definition, within a month is the rule

Although spontaneous resolution of acute eosinophilic pneumonia occur without therapy,patients with Acute eosinophilic pneumonia has more fulminant clinical course . The clinical improvement with corticosteroids is often dramatic, fever and radiographic changes resolve within days and with very little risk of relapse on withdrawal of therapy

The plain radiographic abnormalities in chronic eosinophilic pneumonia reveals patchy, nonsegmental areas of consolidation typically in the mid and upper zones. A distinctive feature in x ray is that the opacities are peripheral and seem to parallel the chest wall (the 'photographic negative of pulmonary oedema')—(G)

40.-----c

This is a case of alveolar proteinosis . Thin-section CT images shows a 'crazy-paving' pattern (made up of a striking geographical distribution of ground-glass opacification and thickened interlobular septa) . Such pattern may be noted in (mucinous) bronchiolo-alveolar carcinoma and exogenous lipoid pneumonia.(G)

41.----a (CHAPTER 25 ,G)

42.-----a (Webb)

43.-----b

LIP does show cysts (Webb)

44.-----a

Abnormalities in asbestosis are usually most severe in the subpleural regions of the lower lobes (Chapter 1,G)

45.-----d

In peri-aortitis, CT shows a thick cuff of enhancing soft tissue around the aorta.(CHAPTER 27 ,G)

46.----a (CHAPTER 6 ,G)

47.-----a

As in conventional angiography, acute embolism is seen as an intravascular filling defect. Contrast medium may be seen to flow around or adjacent to the clot (giving a 'tram track' appearance only if the vessel is in the plane of the image section). (CHAPTER 6 ,G)

48.----e

Approximately 50% of patients with a VSD have an associated additional cardiac abnormality. Coarctation of the aorta and aortic stenosis are particularly important. (CHAPTER 23,G)

49.----e

The prevalence of Eisenmenger syndrome has declined as diagnosis and surgical closure of shunts has greatly improved. (CHAPTER 23 .G)

50.-----b

A normal perfusion scintigraphy excludes acute infarction. (CHAPTER 22,G)

REFERENCES

1.Adam: Grainger & Allison's Diagnostic Radiology, 5th ed.(G)

2.Sutton'sTextbook of Radiology and Imaging, Seventh edition

3. Clinical magnetic resonance imaging.Third edition ,edited by Edelman,Hesselink,Zlatkin an Crues III .Published saunders.

4.CT and MR imaging of the whole body (Haaga)

5.High-Resolution CT of the Lung (Webb)

A consultant radiologist ,**Dr Nagendra Kumar Sinha** has passed MBBS from Patna Medical College and Hospital ,Patna (Bihar ,India) and got his MD (Radiodiagnosis) degree from Assam medical College and Hospital,Dibrugarh (Assam,India).He has worked as DM (Neuroradiology) resident at AIIMS,New Delhi (India).

He is the author of books:

1.FRCR MCQs Physics (MRI and USG) (Amazon.com),

2.MCQs in Radiology (Amazon.com),

3.FRCR PART 1 MCQs RADIOPHYSICS (Amazon.com).

He remains actively involved in different CMEs and conferences .

He administers Nagendra's Radiology Blog (http://nagendraradiology.blogspot.com/) and PATH TO SUCCESS blog (http://nagendraway.blogspot.com/).He has keen interest in personality development and matters of spiritualism.

2

Printed in Great Britain
by Amazon.co.uk, Ltd.,
Marston Gate.